WE CHOOSE TO BE MORE THAN OUR DIAGNOSES

A compilation of stories published by

GUIDING BRILLIANT WRITERS PUBLISHING, LLC

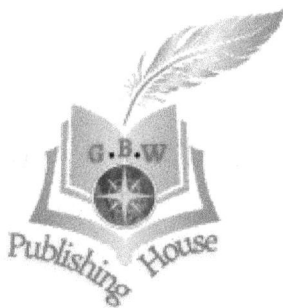

G.B.W

Publishing House

YOU CAN BELIEVE
THE DIAGNOSIS,

NOT THE PROGNOSIS.

~ Deepak Chopra ~

WE CHOOSE…

How we face the kind of life we have been handed.

WE CHOOSE…

Faith over Fear

Love over Anger

Serenity over Antagonism

Our ability to embrace, "ALL" of who we are, including our diagnoses,

is what defines us; not the diagnoses.

Stigma loses its grip when we CHOOSE not to be stigmatized.

I CHOOSE, THEREFORE I AM.

Copyright © 2025 Guiding Brilliant Writers Publishing, LLC. All rights reserved.

The characters and events portrayed in this book are fictitious. Any similarity to real persons, living or dead, is coincidental and not intended by the author. No part of this book may be reproduced, or stored in a retrieval system, or transmitted in any form or by any means, electronic, mechanical, photocopying, recording, or otherwise, without express written permission of the publisher

ISBN: 979-8-9993094-1-9

Cover design by:

GBW Publishing, LLC

Library of Congress Control Number: 2018675309

Printed in the United States of America

Table of Contents

MY DIAGNOSES DON'T DEFINE ME
by Aaron Birn

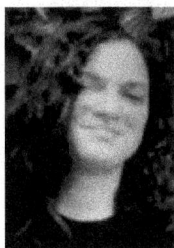

"He has ADHD."

That was the first label placed on me, a simple sentence that would go on to shape much of my childhood and early identity. The diagnosis came after both my parents and many teachers' observations and complaints of me being unable to sit still for extended periods of time and easily losing focus. I was six years old—far too young to fully comprehend what those four letters meant. At that age, I didn't know about brain chemistry, neurodivergence, or how society stigmatizes anything that deviates from the "norm." But I understood one thing very clearly: I was different.

Around the same time as this, my home was constantly filled with shouting—voices raised in anger, sharp words slicing through the walls each night. My parents fought endlessly, over things I didn't understand at the time. As a kid, I thought maybe if I stepped in, if I said the right thing or cried loudly enough, I could stop it. I'd beg them to stop, standing between them like a fragile shield, but it never worked. Eventually, the tension shattered what was left of our family. They got divorced, and everything changed.

After that, my life became a schedule—rigid, court-ordered, and hollow. I was sent back and forth between homes like luggage, never staying long enough to feel settled. Tuesdays and Thursdays after school, I'd be with my dad. Every other weekend too. The rest of the time, I lived with my mom. It was a routine I learned to follow, but it never felt normal. It was like living in two separate worlds, both feeling like home, but only one of them being my actual home.

All the while, I was still trying to make sense of the label that had been pinned to me—ADHD. The chaos at home only amplified the confusion I felt inside. It was hard to tell where the disorder ended and the instability began. Was I restless because of my brain, or because I never knew what version of home I'd be walking into next? I carried that emotional weight into the classroom, even if no one could see it.

In the early years of school, this difference wasn't always visible in the ways adults expected. Sure, I was impulsive and distracted at times, but I was also imaginative and curious. I loved stories and building things, creating complex imaginary worlds in my head and acting them out alone on the playground. The problem was, the classroom had little room for a mind that didn't move in a straight line.

Teachers would call home with concerns: "He won't sit still," "He doesn't focus," "He talks too much," "He seems disorganized." These weren't just observations—they were judgments. Each call chipped away at the idea that I was just a kid trying to learn at my own pace. Instead, I became a problem to fix.

At home, my mom tried her best. She attended meetings, tried routines, read books, and tried to be patient. But frustration would leak through. I saw the weariness in people's eyes when I couldn't finish homework. I felt the disappointment when I blurted things out inappropriately or left a mess in my wake. Even though no one said it directly, the implication hung in the air: Why can't you just behave?

By the time I was eight, I had already internalized the idea that I was too much to handle. That something inside me was inherently broken, unfixable. I began to doubt my worth—not because anyone said it outright, but because of the way people responded to me. The sighs when I asked too many questions, the frustration in teachers' voices, the tension in my teachers' faces when I struggled to sit still or follow directions. I was just a kid, yet already tired of being a burden. I started shrinking myself in ways I didn't fully understand—staying quiet when I wanted to speak, pretending to be fine when I wasn't, trying to be the version of myself I thought others could tolerate. I didn't have the language for it then, but I was already beginning to mask—to hide the parts of me that felt too loud, too chaotic, too much—and in doing so, I started losing sight of who I really was.

Then came age nine—the year everything changed. Not for the better, not yet, but in a way that revealed how complex my struggles truly were.

I stopped going to school.

It started small, with feigning stomach aches, pretending to be too tired, crying quietly in the morning. But it escalated quickly. The anxiety I had always felt—tight in my chest like a coiled spring—erupted. Every morning became a battle of wills between me and my own fear. The idea of school filled me with dread so intense I would freeze. My mom was baffled, then concerned, then desperate. My mom and the school brought in therapists, counselors, even friends to coax me back into the world. Some days it worked. Many days, it didn't.

I didn't have the words to explain what was happening inside me. I just knew everything was too much. The noise of the classroom felt like it was echoing directly into my brain—every pencil tap, every cough, every shifting chair was a spike of discomfort. The pressure to pay attention felt unbearable, like trying to balance on a tightrope while a thousand thoughts pulled me in different directions. I lived in fear of making mistakes, as if one wrong answer or forgotten homework assignment confirmed I wasn't good enough.

And it wasn't just about schoolwork—everything had to be perfect. My behavior. My reactions. My ability to fit in. If it wasn't perfect, it wasn't enough. I couldn't articulate that my mind was racing all the time, tangled up in worst-case scenarios. What if I failed? What if I disappointed someone? What if everyone saw through me and realized I didn't belong? I didn't understand that anxiety had a name, that perfectionism was a shield I'd built to protect myself. I just felt overwhelmed and alone, trapped in a world that moved too fast and expected too much—and no matter how hard I tried, I couldn't keep up.

I didn't know that what I was feeling had a name—anxiety—until a professional finally gave it to me after months of avoidance. When I received that diagnosis, it felt like someone had turned on a light in a dark room. Suddenly, my fear wasn't just "being difficult." It was real, and it had roots. Knowing that didn't make it go away, but it helped. It gave my mom and me a framework to begin healing. But healing is not a straight path; it's messy, full of setbacks and revelations.

Throughout middle school, I walked a fine line between functioning and falling apart. My ADHD was still ever-present. I'd miss assignments, forget materials, and get distracted during lessons. I was always behind, no matter how hard I tried. I missed countless days of school still, even with the diagnosis. My anxiety layered over everything, whispering that failure was inevitable and that people were always judging. I masked it well most days. I'd joke, make people laugh, and try to be the "fun one." But inside, I was often overwhelmed and deeply insecure, to the point that I would wonder if the world would just be better off without me.

With so much already going on, what made things worse was how often I felt misunderstood—especially by the people who were supposed to help. Like my vice principal in middle school, who was convinced I had Oppositional Defiant Disorder simply because I avoided school. He repeated it to my mom like a fact, even when she pushed back and explained that I didn't show any signs of it. They constantly dismissed her—despite her background in psychology, and even more importantly, despite the fact that she was my mother.

Then there was the school psychiatrist at my district high school, someone whose entire job was supposed to center around supporting students' mental health. But instead of listening, she seemed to check boxes. She once handed us a generic behavioral plan with things like "Learn to accept no as an answer." printed on it. All of it was things I already did. She didn't personalize it at all, so we refused to sign. Another time, she asked me if I wanted someone to walk me to my first-period class because I sometimes took a few minutes to get there from the opposite end of the school. I clearly told her no. Imagine my surprise when one morning, a woman showed up, called me by name, and said she'd be walking me to class from now on. I felt completely disregarded—like my voice didn't matter.

When even the professionals—the people meant to advocate for me— couldn't be trusted to listen or care, it left me feeling more isolated than ever. I didn't just feel misunderstood; I felt invisible. With each invalidation, it became harder to know who I could turn to, or if anyone was truly in my corner.

By age 13, the weight of it all began to take a more sinister toll. I didn't want to get out of bed some mornings. I stopped enjoying things that used to make me feel alive. Even talking to friends became exhausting. A kind of numbness set in—a gray fog that dulled everything.

Around this time, the extent of my childhood trauma had started to take a toll on me. When I was young, my father would abuse me. From hitting to yelling, I experienced it all, and up to this point, I thought that was normal. There were times he'd drag me by my legs out of the house to bring me to school or hit me when I tried to stay in his car to spend more time with him after his visitation ended. I thought your parents retaliating whenever you were upset was a thing all kids dealt with, but I finally realised that it wasn't at this age. With this realisation, I felt even more conflicted. I loved my father, but I felt such a deep rooted fear of him that I started to feel an immense guilt about it, but I was still afraid to fully talk about it, so it instead manifested as sadness and depression.

At age 14, I was diagnosed with major depressive disorder.

It was a terrifying but strangely validating moment. Like the previous diagnoses, it gave structure to chaos. Suddenly, the exhaustion, the hopelessness, the inability to feel joy—they weren't signs of weakness. They were symptoms. Treatable. Understandable. Not my fault. For years, I had blamed myself for how I felt. I thought I was lazy, dramatic, or just broken in some invisible way that no one else could see. The diagnosis didn't fix everything overnight, but it gave me something I hadn't had in a long time—language. A name. And most importantly, hope.

At this point, I had been sent to a school specifically for students with mental health challenges because my district decided I was too much to handle. Too unpredictable. Too emotional. Too complicated. It felt like a confirmation of my worst fear: that I wasn't just struggling—I was a problem.

When I first arrived, I felt completely out of place. Nearly everyone there seemed to have more extreme challenges, more visible struggles. Some had been hospitalized, others were dealing with issues I had never encountered before. I spent the first month barely showing up, emotionally shut down and completely disoriented. I missed my friends, my old routines—even the familiarity of the school that had failed me.

But slowly, things started to shift.

I began to see this new school not as a punishment, but as a second chance. An opportunity to prove—to myself and everyone else—that I was capable. That the issue wasn't who I was, but how I'd been treated. I wasn't the failure they thought I was; they had failed to understand me.

So I showed up. I made new friends. I started completing my work, participating in class, asking for help when I needed it. For the first time in a long time, I felt seen for who I actually was—not just my symptoms. I started to build confidence in myself, and I learned strategies to manage the overwhelming thoughts and emotions that had once paralyzed me. I wasn't just surviving anymore—I was growing.

That's not to say the diagnosis and the school transfer fixed everything. It didn't. Depression is not like a cold you recover from with rest. It's more like a shadow—sometimes long and dark, sometimes barely visible, but always lurking. But knowing its name allowed me to fight it. I was no longer swinging in the dark—I had a target, something to face head-on.

Despite having been in therapy most of my life, this was when therapy really began to change things for me. Not because my therapist had suddenly become wiser or more skilled, but because I was finally ready to do the hard work. I wasn't just there because someone told me to be—I was there for myself. I began learning actual coping mechanisms: grounding techniques for when I felt overwhelmed, cognitive reframing for the negative thoughts that swirled around endlessly, and mindfulness strategies that helped me stay connected to the present.

I also started looking inward. I had to. It was painful—like ripping off old scabs just to let wounds breathe. I began confronting deeply rooted fears: my fear of being abandoned, my compulsive need to be perfect, and this pervasive belief that I simply wasn't enough. Therapy forced me to question those beliefs. Where did they come from? Who planted them in me, and why had I watered them for so long?

One of the most pivotal points in my healing came the following year. I finally found the courage to talk about the abuse I had endured— something I had kept buried under shame and confusion. With support, I confronted it head-on. I reached a tipping point when my father, in one final act of control, breached my privacy and tried to undermine my relationship with my mother. That was it. I cut him out of my life completely.

It hurt. Deeply. Cutting off a parent isn't just a decision—it's a grief process. But the pain was honest, and for the first time, it was mine. I chose it. And I chose peace over chaos.

He denied everything, of course. Denied the abuse, denied the breach of trust. But that no longer mattered. His validation was no longer required for my healing. My well-being didn't hinge on someone else's denial, especially not his.

Through this process, I learned something powerful: emotions are not the enemy. I had spent so long afraid of them, trying to numb them, outrun them, bury them. But they weren't the problem. They were messengers. I began to see crying not as weakness, but as release. I learned that sometimes growth feels like heartbreak. Sometimes choosing yourself means walking away from the people who made you.

Even now, years later, I carry the weight of those decisions. There's still a lingering sense of disconnect from my peers. They spent three years building memories together in high school while I was somewhere else, navigating my own private storm. Now, they're off at college, moving forward, while I sometimes feel like I'm still catching up. There are moments where I feel like an outsider in my own friends group. Like I missed a chapter of life I was supposed to live.

But here's what I've come to understand—they want me around. Not because of the experiences I missed, but because of who I am now. They don't see me as broken or behind. They see me. And being loved for who

I am, not what I've been through, is one of the most healing experiences of all.

The most important realization I've had is that I am not my diagnoses. I have ADHD. I have anxiety. I have depression. But they do not define me. They explain parts of me, sure—why I sometimes spiral, why my mind races, why I get overwhelmed—but they are not the whole of me.

And yet, for so long, I believed they were. I believed that being "too much" meant I could never be enough. I believed that struggling made me weak. I believed that if anyone saw the chaos inside my head, they would walk away, but I was wrong.

I've learned that vulnerability is strength. My story, the good, the bad, and the ugly parts, are worth telling. There's power in surviving. There's power in showing up when everything in you wants to disappear. There's power in saying, "I'm still here."

Today, I'm still on this journey. I have bad days. I still get stuck in spirals. I still wrestle with self-doubt and hopelessness. Sometimes, it feels like my mind is holding a trial, trying to figure out which diagnosis is responsible for me feeling poorly. Other times I feel my subconscious judging every decision I make, telling me that I'm a failure. There are still days where I don't want to get out of bed, where I don't want to put energy into anything.

Even in those dark moments, when everything feels heavy and my thoughts turn against me, there's a quiet voice that reminds me of how far I've come. It doesn't always shout, sometimes it's only a whisper, but it's there. It reminds me that pain doesn't erase progress, that healing doesn't mean I never hurt again. It just means I know how to face the hurt differently now. Where I once felt powerless, I've built a foundation—messy, imperfect, but mine—that I can lean on. And that makes all the difference.

But I also have tools. I have people. I have resilience. And I've learned to celebrate small victories like getting out of bed on a tough day, finishing a project I've avoided, asking for help when I need it, saying "no" when I don't want to do something.

Despite everything, I am genuinely happy with where I am. Not because my life is perfect, but because I've fought hard for the peace I have now. Every scar tells a story, not of defeat, but of survival. And I've learned something else—something I want everyone who's ever felt like me to hear:

There is nothing wrong with you. You are not a failure because your brain works differently. You are not weak because you feel deeply. It's ok to reach out and ask for help from people when you're hurting, in fact, the courage it takes to do that is commendable. You are not broken because life has been hard, you are exactly who you're supposed to be.

The world isn't always built for people like us. It's built for order, predictability, compliance—for quiet minds that follow straight lines. But we don't fit into neat boxes, and that doesn't make us broken. It makes us different. It makes us powerful in ways the world doesn't always recognize. We are creative—we see connections others miss. We are adaptive—we've had to be, navigating systems that weren't designed with us in mind. We are emotionally intelligent—not in spite of our struggles, but because of them. And we are strong—stronger than anyone knows, because we've survived things no one can see just by looking at us.

I am more than my ADHD.

I am more than my anxiety.

I am more than my depression.

I am a son. A friend. A learner. A survivor. A thinker. A fighter.

I am a work in progress, and that is enough.

I am allowed to be both a masterpiece and a mess at the same time.

And I will not let my past define my future.

Healing isn't easy. It isn't quick. It isn't linear. Some days it looks like joy, like breakthroughs, like peace. Other days, it looks like getting out of bed when everything hurts, or forgiving yourself for falling short, but it is possible. It takes patience. It takes honesty. It takes courage to sit with discomfort instead of running from it. And above all, it takes compassion, not just for yourself but also others. Because we're all fighting battles people can't see.

So if you're reading this and you're struggling, let me say it again—you are not alone. Your pain is real. Your feelings are valid. Your story is not over. There is hope, even when you can't see it. There is strength in simply making it to tomorrow.

Keep going. The world needs people like us—people who feel deeply, who fight hard, who notice the little things, who bring color to gray spaces. People who carry scars but keep showing up. People who turn their pain into purpose.

You matter.

You are enough.

You are still becoming.

And that is something worth holding onto.

BIO:

Aaron Birn is a creative and passionate young adult making his publishing debut with We Choose to Be More Than Our Diagnosis. Aaron has always expressed himself through singing, dancing, drawing, painting, and digital design. His love for video games goes beyond playing—he dreams of developing games, characters, and marketing campaigns in the industry.

A talented graphic artist, Aaron's artwork was regularly selected for high school exhibits. His favorite subjects have always been art and music. He is expanding his skills through an internship with Uniqua Beauty Norm, and its founder, Jenlyn Ford, where he combines his creativity with marketing, branding, and design.

Aaron lives by the belief that he is more than his diagnoses of ADHD, Social Anxiety, and Major Depressive Disorder. Having often been misunderstood by parts of society, throughout his childhood, he is determined to advocate for others while showing the world that people with diagnoses are whole, talented, and capable human beings.

When people meet Aaron, he hopes they see his kindness, humor, creativity, and compassion first—his diagnoses are part of his journey, but they do not define him. Aaron is proud to use his voice in this anthology to inspire others to see beyond labels and recognize the incredible potential within every individual.

Aaron also enjoys cooking, spending time with his mom, playing games with friends, watching YouTube videos, and hanging out with his best friend, Minnie, the family's rescued Lab-mix.

HOW I LEARNED TO FLY
by Crystal Behe

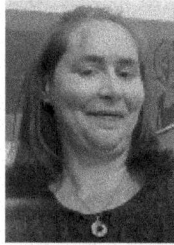

Do you ever feel like you hide parts of yourself from others, like you hide your dog's meds in a piece of cheese? That's how I felt for most of my life. Mental health was non-existent in my house growing up. When it was brought up, it was always in hushed tones like a dirty secret that shouldn't be let out. This mindset has affected me throughout my life more than I ever realized. It wasn't until I was 37 years old and recently out of a very abusive relationship that I found a therapist who actually saw me and correctly diagnosed me with A.D.H.D., C.P.T.S.D., and neurodivergence. I sometimes wonder what would be different if I had been properly diagnosed as a teenager, how different my life would have been.

As a kid, I remember my mom never talking about anything related to negative feelings. She looked down on medicines like Adderall and Ritalin, making comments like "Now he's just a zombie. She should be able to control him without drugging him." It felt like she was saying that mental disabilities like A.D.H.D., anxiety, depression, and the like weren't real, and that the parents are to blame for not being stricter with their kids. When I was in eighth grade, and was forced to go to therapy by the Department of Children and Families, to get help regarding my home life, she made a mockery of it by finding a therapist who could be bought. That instilled a distrust of therapy in me, which was reinforced when I was 17, and in a program for troubled teens. They tried to diagnose me with borderline personality disorder, which was way off base. I will get into that in a bit.

It wasn't until recently that I found out why my mom felt the way she does about mental disabilities. It was because of her upbringing; her mom had been in and out of mental institutions her entire childhood, because of what she went through during World War 2. I think she grew up feeling ashamed and blamed her mom, for the things lacking in her life, and the fact that she had to be the mom to her two younger siblings. I genuinely believe it's because of this that she has what I call, the ostrich syndrome, you know, burying your head in the sand until whatever is wrong goes away. She never wanted to hurt me; she didn't understand that she was a victim of generational trauma, and in turn, continuing the cycle. I have spoken with her in-depth about this in the last few years, and we have made peace with what happened while I was growing up. It's tough because life is messy, and so is generational dysfunction, abuse, & lack of emotional intelligence, wellness, and safety.

The thing is, the signs were all there about me having adhd, but back then, it was just a boy's diagnosis, not girls. I would talk too much in class, get easily distracted, and get bored with subjects I didn't like. I also had difficulty memorizing some things, but could remember a book I read months or years prior. So, by not having me tested for neurodivergence and adhd in my youth, my education and life were very much altered from what they should have been. Having a proper diagnosis allows you to learn how to work with it, and recognize the signs, and what to do to embrace and live with it.

Now that I have covered the lack of proper mental health diagnosis within my home, let's discuss the misdiagnosis that was attempted to be given to me by my counselor in the youth program I was in. Now I will say that when I was told about this, my mom took me to the bookstore, and we bought a few books on it. This is what we found. Borderline Personality Disorder (BPD) typically isn't diagnosed until a person is in their mid-20s because of how the human brain, and personality, develop during adolescence and early adulthood - definitely not at 17.

Here's why:
1. Personality is Still Forming
In teens and young adults, identity, emotional regulation, and behavior patterns are still maturing. What may appear as symptoms of BPD—such as emotional instability, impulsiveness, or intense relationships—can be a regular part of adolescent development.

2. The Brain is Still Developing
The prefrontal cortex, which controls decision-making, impulse regulation, and emotional reasoning, continues to develop into the mid-20s. Some traits that resemble BPD may resolve naturally as the brain matures.

3. Risk of Misdiagnosis
Early symptoms of BPD can overlap with other conditions (like depression, anxiety, trauma response, or ADHD), which can lead to incorrect labeling, and inappropriate treatment, if diagnosed too early.
4. Stigma and Identity Concerns

Labeling a teen with a personality disorder can affect their self-identity and mental health trajectory, reinforcing a sense of being "broken" or "permanently disordered" during a fragile developmental phase.

Armed with this information, my mom had me transferred to the other counselor in the program, especially because the woman who tried to diagnose me wasn't even a licensed therapist. The thing is, it made me even more untrusting of mental health professionals, and it stayed with me until long into my twenties. Which is ironic as my aunt always said I would be an excellent therapist because of my natural empathic nature, wanting to help people, and outgoing personality. I did take some psychology classes during my first attempt at college, when I thought I wanted to be a teacher, thinking it would help me when working with my students and their parents.

Now let's move forward to my mid thirties when I started thinking that therapy might be needed, and that not all therapists are like what I experienced as a child, the memory would resurface about the child therapist. She'd helped me when I was 7 years old, to deal with the nightmares I was having, she was kind and did help. At first, it was because I wanted my now ex-partner to go to therapy for his anger issues, along with both of us together for family therapy, but he refused. When I finally left him, my mental state was in shambles, and I bit the bullet, and went to both addiction and mental health therapy. This is when I was formally diagnosed with C.P.T.S.D., A.D.H.D., and, because of the physical trauma to my brain from the abuse I endured - neurodivergent. She asked me why I was never diagnosed with ADHD and also why no one helped me with my issues from my childhood, and well, I have already explained that to you, my dear reader. But getting this diagnosis put a lot of my life and personality traits into perspective for me. It also made me realise that if I had been correctly diagnosed, how different my life would have been.

You see, the thing about being properly diagnosed is that you learn how to work with it, instead of not understanding why you are acting the way you are. As I continued with my therapy and putting my life back together after the shambles it was from my bad choices, I began finding ways to cope and improve myself. Recognizing the things that trigger my anxiety, a side effect of my C.P.T.S.D., and how to recognize when my focus is slipping due to my A.D.H.D., are just a few things that have helped. I began researching all three of my diagnoses, wanting to understand them better, trying all different types of therapies and coping tools, and have able to come up with a toolbox that works for me. I have made a support system of tools, and amazing people who help me when I am struggling, and acknowledge when I have made breakthroughs and growth.

It has been almost five years since I was diagnosed correctly, and I am still working through the traumas that caused the CPTSD and neurodivergence. I was watching one of my favorite comedians, Taylor Tomlinson, the other day, and when she was talking about her own diagnosis of bipolar, and what happened, it really resonated with me. During the show, when she said she told her therapist that she didnt know how she felt about it, she said her therapist responded with, "Well, you can always say, 'I have bi-polar, not I am bi-polar,' and I said isn't that like saying, You are acting like a bitch?" And that part really made me both laugh and think about it. I think she is right in the sense that being something doesn't have to define you. As someone who has multiple mental health diagnoses, I agree that they don't define me, but they are a part of who I am. The little personality quirks are a result of different aspects of each diagnosis. For example, the way I can go from point A to point Z when in a conversation, a talent I call the "7 degrees to Kevin Bacon mindset", some people understand it, while others, I usually have to explain how I got there. Also, how I don't like it when people feel the need to over-explain things to me, as if I can't understand their point when they made it, yet I tend to over-explain because of my self-esteem issues, something that I have been overcoming slowly. I multitask and prefer to have something that keeps my mind and hands busy, and I am the most extroverted introvert you will ever meet. All of these are results of my diagnosis, but I use them in different ways in both my professional, and personal life.

I won't lie that there are times where it is easier just to say "I have adhd or am neuro-spicy" to explain my actions to someone who doesn't know me, or as a joke with others who are showing signs of the same, like adhd. I also use them to break the ice when speaking with people about my calling. But I don't use it as a way to define myself. I refuse to be put in this tiny box that is characterized by my mental "disabilities", especially considering they aren't the only part of my personality that shines through. My ability to empathize with others, my loyalty, and ability to problem solve and mediate issues, along with my natural leadership ability, are not causes of my mental disabilities, but core parts of my personality.

Over the years, I have dabbled in many different ideas for my career, never settling on anything, another characteristic of my ADHD, but one thing was a constant: I always wanted to be of service in some way. After I was in therapy for a while, I finally made the choice I fought for years; I am going back to school to get my psychology degree, to be able to truly help others like myself. I refuse to live by labels and what society claims I am, whether it is my mental health diagnosis or domestic abuse victim, as these are not who I am. Yes, they are a part of me, but it is because of them and the rest of my life experiences that I can work with the people I do. I can help them because at some point or another in my life, I was them, and have the tools to be able to help them break out of the boxes that they are in. To let them know that they aren't alone, and aren't broken or flawed because they have a disability or trauma, they just have different abilities that should be embraced, and used to lift themselves up, and learn how to navigate life with confidence. I am Crystal "Phoenix" Behe, and choose to fly using my diagnosis as the wind beneath my wings, not to break them.

BIO:

Crystal Behe is a passionate advocate, speaker, and survivor dedicated to empowering others who have experienced domestic violence and abuse. As someone who has walked the painful path of healing, Crystal knows firsthand the courage it takes to reclaim your voice and identity after trauma. Diagnosed with chronic post-traumatic stress disorder (C-PTSD), anxiety, and ADHD, she shares her journey with raw honesty and unwavering strength in We Are More Than Our Diagnosis.

Crystal's mission is deeply personal: to provide survivors with the space and support they need to share their stories in their own words, on their terms. Through her work, she offers practical strategies, emotional support, and access to vital resources to help survivors move from victimhood to empowerment. She believes every survivor deserves to be heard, seen, and supported as they step into their truth and embrace their resilience.

In her chapter, Crystal sheds light not only on the realities of living with invisible diagnoses but also offers hope, reminding readers that healing is possible—and that they are never alone.

www.youtube.com/@CrystalPhoenix8320
www.riseofcrystalphoenix.com

THE QUIET POWER OF BEING SEEN
by Crystal Chilcott-Ruzycki

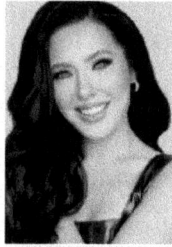

When I was about to graduate from college, I received a job offer to coach figure skating in Iceland. I had to move nine days after graduating from college, so I got my diploma and flew to Iceland. I knew no one there and I thought my adventure of living in the land of the midnight sun and northern lights was going to be my big adventure. I had no idea a type 1 diabetes diagnosis awaited me there.

The shift happened quickly. Going from being young and healthy to living with one of the world's oldest, deadliest, and most misunderstood diseases happened practically overnight. After a couple of weeks of extreme thirst and fatigue, and rapid weight loss, I knew it was time to seek a diagnosis. I knew something was wrong, but nobody would believe me. I tried to get the information about how to access a doctor in Iceland. I kept looking up information online about my symptoms. When I Googled it, I discovered that I had every single symptom of diabetes.

When I did finally go to the doctor, he dismissed my concerns, saying the swollen ankles were just from standing in my skates all week. I said that I Googled my symptoms and wanted to get bloodwork done at least. They agreed. The next day, I got a phone call that my blood sugar was three times the normal number. I had to immediately go to the diabetes center in Reykjavik, where they ran a C-petide test to confirm that it was indeed type 1 and not type 2. The misconception that type 1 diabetes is only diagnosed in childhood persists and many adults are misdiagnosed as type 2. A C-peptide test shows the level of insulin product and assists in the diagnosis of type 1 diabetes. I was fortunate that the doctor didn't think type 2 was likely given my lifestyle and ordered the test

I was given two types of insulin, told that I had type 1 diabetes, and that my whole life was going to change. They showed me how to check my blood sugar. I needed to prick my finger on a meter, which measured my blood sugar, then compare it to what they told me was normal. Mine was way too high, despite fasting. The proof was right there. The betrayal came from my own body which I had previously trusted to take me across the stage and ice, and on flights to distant countries, but now it seemed like a stranger I couldn't trust.

I also noticed right away how people started to treat me differently. One morning, I arrived at the rink for coaching early and was putting on my skates near the ice. One of the other coaches came downstairs and said, "I didn't see you in the lounge so I was so worried something happened to you with your blood sugar!" It wasn't the concern that bothered me, it was that everyone had started to see me as my diagnosis. That same coach came over the day after my diagnosis, and as she was making coffee in my kitchen, she asked, "I don't suppose you have any sugar do you? Of course you wouldn't, you're diabetic." I didn't, in fact, have sugar in my kitchen, but that was because I drank my coffee and tea without sweetener before my diagnosis. At this point, I had only known I was diabetic for two days. This incident showed me something else I thought was strange. Some people seemed to think I somehow always knew I'd be diabetic and that I would have accepted my diagnosis right away.

Type 1 Diabetes is shrouded in misconceptions, outdated science, and casual cruelty. Most of the public and even medical knowledge is either outdated or inaccurate. Despite changing the name from "juvenile" to "type 1 diabetes," the misconception that type 1 is only diagnosed in childhood continues. This is demonstrably false. Over half of new cases are diagnosed in adults, with some estimates as high as 60%. There is also another idea that in order to be diagnosed, you have to have a family history of the disease. While there may be a genetic component, this is also another misconception: over 90% of new cases have no family history of the disease. The exact cause of type 1 is still unknown, but it is likely a mix of genetic and environmental factors. It is not caused by diet or lifestyle. The comments of, "Did you eat a lot of sugar as a kid?" or posting a photo of a dessert and saying "#diabetes" further increases the stigma. One of the most frustrating things early on in my diagnosis was when a drink called a "unicorn iced latte" came out full of sugar and my social media feeds were full of comments like, "fast-track to diabetic coma" and "guess we're all getting diabetes now." Even people who prided themselves on supporting those living with chronic illnesses or disabilities, often "forgot" that diabetes isn't a punchline to a joke. When telling a friend about this, she said, "People just don't understand. They don't really mean that." I responded that this was exactly the problem.

When I was first diagnosed, well-meaning, but misinformed people started to tell me all the things I couldn't do anymore: travel, compete on stage in a pageant, or eat certain foods. None of these things were true.

I also got a lot of unsolicited advice about diabetes management. A common piece of advice I received was, "get an insulin pump." There's an idea out there that an insulin pump does everything for the diabetic. You plug it in and never have to think about it again. This couldn't be further from the truth. An insulin pump comes with its own set of challenges: technology failures, changing them every three days to a new site, and, like with taking insulin injections, requires manually inputting the number of carbs at each meal.

With a new diagnosis of type 1 diabetes, there is usually a "honeymoon phase" where the body is still making some insulin, but at unpredictable intervals. Because of this and because an insulin pump requires a certain minimum amount of insulin per day, I was not recommended to go on a pump right away.

About six years into my diagnosis, I started using an Omnipod, a tubeless insulin pump. I also use a CGM or continuous glucose monitor. The continuous glucose monitor sends my blood sugar number to my phone and also communicates with my pump to know how much basal or background insulin to give. I have to put on a new pump every three days and a new CGM every ten days.

When I was diagnosed, I was an active participant in the Miss America pageant system. Pageantry has been a part of my life since I was 9 years old, when I first competed in some local and festival pageants. As I grew older, I was increasingly drawn to the community service aspect of pageantry, and that is something that continues to this day. I realized that I could use my platform, and voice within pageantry, as a way of advocating for others living with diabetes or other invisible illnesses.

I stood in my new evening gown and started thinking about where I would wear my insulin pump and continuous glucose monitor. Someone shopping with me turned to me and said, "With a gown this beautiful, you shouldn't ruin it with a pump." That made me realize that there was still a lot of work that needed to be done. Instead of trying to hide my insulin pump, I ordered a custom designed sticker to match the beading of my gown. Wearing a swimsuit and gown on stage was daunting at first, but I started to make so many connections because of being open about it.

When I got married, I decided to keep my pageantry journey going by competing for the title of Mrs. Colorado. I was on my way to my very first event, a sustainable clothing fashion show, when I realized how exposed and obvious my insulin pump was on my arm. I started to wonder if I should have worn something that covered it up. As soon as I walked in the door, a woman came up to me and asked, "Is that an Omnipod?" I replied that it was and she told me that she worked for the company that helped develop the insulin pump. She was so excited to see a patient with one "out in the wild" and could show it to her daughter. At another event, I walked in to judge a pageant for children and teenagers. One of the teen contestants also had an Omnipod on her arm and was so excited to see an adult with a pump as well.

Living with diabetes can be isolating because of the misconceptions and the stigma, but we are never alone. The moment I chose visibility, I found something I didn't expect: connection, community, and the quiet power of being seen.

BIO:

Crystal Chilcott-Ruzycki was diagnosed with type 1 diabetes when she was 23 years old and coaching figure skating in Iceland. Going from being young and healthy to living with one of the world's oldest, deadliest, and most misunderstood diseases, practically overnight made it difficult at first not to feel defined by her diagnoses. Instead of asking her, "How are you?" People would ask her, "What's your blood sugar?" She then made a conscious decision not to let her diagnosis define her and wrote Gliding on Insulin about a type 1 diabetic figure skater to help inspire children that they are not just their diagnosis. Breaking the stigma around this disease and inspiring other diabetics is her mission. When she is not writing or advocating for diabetes, she enjoys spending time with her husband, Brian, her two cats, two turtles, and ten fish tanks. She also enjoys traveling and has been to 33 countries.

www.facebook.com/crystal.chilcott
www.facebook.com/crystal.chilcott

THE DAY I ASKED GOOGLE IF MY HUSBAND WOULD GET THE LIFE INSURANCE

by Deb Haas

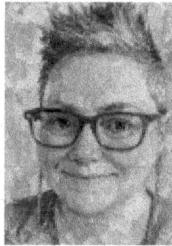

It didn't start with a diagnosis.

It started with a bottle of sleeping pills and a question.

Not a dramatic question. Not shouted into the void.

It was quiet. Curious. Practically clinical.

I wonder what would happen if I took all 30 of these?

That was the question.

And the answer?

Nothing.

Not emotionally, anyway.

I didn't feel panic.

Or fear.

Or sadness.

I didn't feel anything.

That was the scariest part.

So I did what any high-functioning, burnt-out, emotionally stunted woman with a 24-year career in corporate HR might do: I Googled it.

If I die by suicide, will my husband still get the life insurance payout?

(The answer, by the way, is yes - if the policy is over two years old.)

I remember thinking, People say if you're serious, you don't tell anyone. You just do it.

And then, barely a whisper, a thought came through:

Deb, it should concern you that you don't feel anything about this choice. That you're treating it like deciding whether or not to go to the store.

That voice saved my life.

The Cracks That Came Before

It hadn't always been this way.

Or maybe it had - but I'd become very good at masking.

The pandemic years were brutal.

Between 2020 and 2023, I lost people I loved. Quietly. Inwardly. The kind of grief that doesn't scream, but reshapes you in silence.

At the same time, my body was rebelling. Menopause hit like a freight train. I wasn't sleeping - maybe two or three hours a night, with sleeping pills. I'd go full nights without rest, just a vibrating hum of anxiety I couldn't shut off.

That April - less than a month into Minnesota's lockdown - I had a telemedicine visit and asked my doctor about relief for the hot flashes. She listed a few medications. When she got to the one that could help with both menopause symptoms and anxiety, I started crying.

Not because I was sad.

Because I finally felt seen.

She didn't judge. Just said gently,

"Looks like that's the one. I'll write the prescription today."

That moment planted a seed.

But the burnout? That still had more room to grow.

I finally got the promotion I'd desired for years in December 2022. And it was almost like, having reached that longed-for point, I started to crash.

Then in January 2023, some people who'd been with the company were laid off with no fanfare. No recognition of decades of service. And some part of me knew what was coming.

From that point, my work started slipping. I started spacing on attending calls. I was late all the time - when before, I'd made a point of being early.

Not doing my work. Burying myself in TV, books, games - anything that felt better than being crappy at my job.

And then my 90-year-old father passed away unexpectedly at the end of May 2023. I'd driven up to see him the day before. We made sammiches and had a lovely talk. He even shared some things from his history I'd never known.

The next day, I got a panicked call from my brother - Dad was on the floor, paramedics trying to revive him.

Looking back, that was the final straw for my burnout.

I planned the entire funeral - the music, the readings, every detail. I kept my two warring brothers from raging at each other. I pulled it off, telling myself over and over: I don't have time to grieve.

Then a week later, my husband picked up my monthly prescription for sleeping pills. I opened the bottle. Looked down at those 30 little pills. And thought, I wonder what would happen if I took all 30 of these?

And it was an honest question. I felt nothing.

So I slept my usual 2 hours that night. Gave my husband a kiss when he came in to say goodbye on his way to work. Picked up my phone and Googled whether he'd still get the life insurance if I killed myself.

Later that same day - during my very first session with a BetterUp coach - I told them what I'd done and asked if I should consider requesting a leave of absence (LOA) from work. I felt guilty even asking. Convinced there was something wrong with me.

But I did ask. And that was the start.

My LOA officially started the week of July 4th. I entered a partial hospitalization program at the end of July and stayed in treatment for 10 days.

I returned to work on September 1, 2023. That same day, my boss's boss informed me that my layoff date would be March 1, 2024.

Diagnosis: Powered by Impulse, Deductible, and Sheer Determination

It wasn't until November 2024 - after more than six months of unemployment, after finally landing a contract gig in September and fending off the wolves at the door - that I had the moment.

Smidge and I were on our way to dinner. I was in the passenger seat, scrolling through my phone, watching an ADHD video a friend had sent. The creator was acting out funny, painfully accurate examples of ADHD overthinking - and how it looks to everyone else.

As we parked and I walked around the back of the car, I looked at Smidge and said, "Do you think I might have ADHD?"

Smidge didn't miss a beat. He just looked at me with that classic deadpan face and said, "Ah, DUH."

Thanks to my particular brand of impulsive ADHD - and the hard-earned lesson that if I wanted something done, I needed to act on it immediately - I went home that night and logged into MyChart. I messaged my primary care doctor (the one I will go to until she retires or I die, whichever comes first) and asked for a referral to get tested.

They told me the ADHD evaluation typically took multiple days, and their office was nearly 50 miles away. But I had already hit my insurance deductible for the year thanks to my partial hospitalization - and the clock was ticking. If I wanted the whole thing covered, I had to move.

Fast.

So I did what I always do: I committed.

I scheduled the full battery of tests for a single day - over six hours of continuous testing. IQ, memory, puzzles, visual processing, auditory sequencing, attention assessments, you name it. And I loved it.

Seriously. I had a blast. Even the boring tests. Even the ones most people dread. I was chipper, energized, locked in. Every time the psychologist asked if I wanted a break, I'd grin and say, "Nope, let's go!"

When I returned on December 24, 2024, for the results - because I needed to get the visit in before the end of the year and work around the holidays - she asked me how I felt during testing. I told her the truth: I had a great time. I could've kept going.

She smiled, a little wearily, and said, "I was so exhausted by the end of testing you, I had to go home and isolate."

The Day It Had a Name

On December 24, 2024 - Christmas Eve - I got the results.
When she gave me the results, I don't remember much of what she said after it. Because one phrase swallowed the room:

With executive function deficits.
Those four words echoed in my head, so loud and consuming that I can't recall the rest of the visit - or even the drive home.
I hadn't prepared for that combination.
I knew ADHD was likely. I'd done the research. Watched the videos.
But executive function deficits?
That sounded… permanent.

Damaged.

Broken.

It confirmed the fear I had never said out loud:

That there really was something wrong with me.

I went home and disappeared into my cave - my bedroom, my lair, my escape hatch.

Crawled under a blanket and hit play on Twilight.

Yes, that Twilight. Sparkly vampires and teenage melodrama.

It wasn't about quality - it was about hiding. About familiarity. About numbing.

That's when the shame hit.

Not the loud, sobbing kind. The quiet, seeping kind. The kind that whispers:

You can never tell anyone this.

Just say you have ADHD. Leave the rest out.

Nobody needs to know about the broken parts.

I opened ChatGPT and started typing questions. Anything to make the words sound less final. Less loaded. Less... shameful.

But they didn't go away.

They still haven't.

What's changed is this:

I stopped letting them make me small.

The next morning, I did something I never thought I'd do.

I told people.

I shared the whole thing - not just the ADHD, but the executive function deficits too.

Because the truth is, mental health stigma doesn't disappear when we hide.

It disappears when we name it.

When we let people see the whole picture - even the parts we thought made us unlovable.

My perspective had been shaped by the generation that raised me.

My parents were from the Silent Generation. My own GenX cohort was taught to handle things quietly, privately, often with a heaping side of shame.

But I'm done with that.

If someone sees my story and it helps them feel less alone, more curious, more empowered to ask questions - then sharing it is worth it.

I choose transparency.

I choose light.

I choose truth over stigma.

And I choose joy - every messy, marvelous day of it.

After the Diagnosis: Making Peace With My Brain

The diagnosis didn't fix anything.

It didn't suddenly make me more focused or organized or able to remember why I walked into a room. It didn't reconnect me to the part of myself I'd ignored for most of my life - the emotional center I'd learned to skip over entirely. Thoughts? Check. Actions? Always. But feelings? I'd left those out of the loop for decades.

But it did change everything.

Because now I had language.

I had context.

I had a map - and for the first time, I wasn't gaslighting myself about how hard the terrain had been.

I stopped trying to out-perform my so-called flaws.

I started asking for what I needed.

Like visuals. Written plans. Calendars with times attached, not vague "sometime this week" nonsense that used to float away on the breeze. I began to see the patterns - that I live in two zones: Now and Not Now. If it's not Now, it needs a system or it disappears.

And the shame? It didn't vanish. But it lost its grip.

I started hearing the voice that used to berate me for forgetting things or interrupting people or missing deadlines - and I didn't believe it anymore. I could recognize it without absorbing it.

I talked less and listened more. I let my husband finish his sentences. I stopped filling every silence with humor or noise just to prove I was valuable.

Because I started believing I was valuable even when I wasn't producing.

Even when I wasn't entertaining.

Even when I was just... being.

I gave myself permission to speak up when my brain did something beautifully weird. I let the "wild ideas" come out of my mouth instead of stuffing them back in. And I watched people light up when they saw what I saw - or at the very least, when they felt seen by me.

That's what changed.

I didn't become a new person.

I finally became myself.

More Than a Diagnosis: Building a Life That Fits Me

I didn't set out to build a business.

I set out to save my life.

After the diagnosis, the layoff, the grief, the burnout, and the slow climb back to myself - I realized something:

I couldn't go back.

Not to the version of me that over-functioned to survive.

Not to the career ladder that looked more like a treadmill.

Not to shrinking, silencing, or shaping myself into something more digestible for corporate comfort.

So I built The Unexamined Mind.

Not as a polished brand, but as a living, breathing declaration:

I am more than what broke me.

I am more than how I masked.

I am more than my diagnosis.

I work differently now.

I rest more. I write publicly. I speak loudly - and sometimes off-key, because I'm singing again, too. I create spaces for other people like me - the sparkle-hearted misfits, the brain-weird rebels, the deeply feeling doers who are tired of pretending to be fine.

I don't have a 5-year plan.

I have a compass.

And it points toward joy.

Not toxic positivity - but real, grounded, wild joy.

The kind that says, You don't have to earn your worth.

The kind that says, This gets to be fun.

The kind that makes room for tears and laughter in the same breath.

I still have executive function issues.

I still forget things.

I still interrupt when I get excited.

And I still sometimes spiral into the not-enoughness of being human in a world that rewards the performance of perfection.

But I am here.

Fully.

Finally.

And if you're reading this - if you've ever wondered whether your brain is broken, whether you're too much or not enough, whether you'll ever find a way to make your life fit - let me tell you:

You're not broken.

You're not behind.

You're not alone.

You're on the edge of something new.

And it's not too late to choose differently.

To choose truth.

To choose joy.

To choose yourself.
I did.
And I'm not going back.

BIO:

Deb Haas spent over two decades navigating corporate HR with compassion, clarity, and the uncanny ability to make sense of organizational chaos. But in 2024, nine months after being laid off from the company where she'd spent most of her career, she was diagnosed with ADHD. Suddenly, the decades of procrastinating on boring tasks (and feeling like a failure because of it) made a whole lot more sense.

Rather than crawl back into the corporate world with a tidy narrative and a freshly updated résumé, Deb did what any curious, creative, slightly-rebellious Gen Xer might do: she started something weird and wonderful. Her business, The Unexamined Mind, helps people - especially midlife women and recovering perfectionists - reclaim joy, curiosity, and a sense of possibility at work and in life.

She teaches people how to use AI tools in deeply human ways, creates communities that blend play with purpose, and writes a satirical HR newsletter called 404: HR Not Found that's as insightful as it is irreverent. Deb lives in Minneapolis, MN with her husband and three cats, all of whom are excellent at interrupting her flow state. She believes ADHD isn't a deficit - it's a different operating system. One that runs on interest, urgency, and the occasional glitter-fueled breakthrough.

This chapter is her reminder (to herself and others) that diagnoses don't define us - but they can help us understand ourselves more clearly than we ever imagined.

THE UNSPOKEN LESSONS
by Brian Bothe aka Jack Torrance

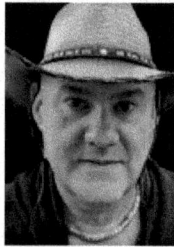

It was the beginning of sixth grade, in the fluorescent-lit halls of Marstellar Middle School in Manassas, Virginia, that I began to understand something quietly brutal: I was not like the others. I wasn't slower or stupid—though that would become the common refrain. I was simply... misaligned. The world moved in straight lines. I curled inward.

This was the early 1980s, and the world was not built for the sensitive. Not for the different. Not for boys who struggled to read aloud or whose teeth jutted out like a punchline. Back then, the words "learning disability" were rarely spoken aloud, and when they were, they carried shame like a stench. There was no vocabulary yet for neurodivergence. Just labels. Lazy. Trouble. Disruption. There was no kindness in the system—only corridors of shame, echoing with laughter that cut like broken glass cutting into my veins of sensitivity and delicacy.

I don't remember all my teachers' names—memory blurs the ordinary. But pain brands its own. Let's call her Mrs. Flanagan. She taught sixth grade English. Her voice was mild, timid even, but when it summoned my name to read aloud, it felt like thunder. But in front of twenty-five, or thirty other kids, it sounded like a sentence. A summoning.

Mrs. Flanagan's sixth grade English became a hellish nightmare for a sensitive kid like me when I was called on to read out loud. My heart would punch against my ribs like it wanted out. The black print on the page looked like ants crawling, blurring, rearranging themselves into riddles only other kids could solve.

As she called out my name to read aloud, her tone was gentle, but her words hit me like a hammer. I stared at the paragraph on page forty-two or maybe it was page one hundred forty-two. I knew where the words started, but by the time my lips moved, the sentence had already unraveled in my brain. The page was nearly a total blur before me. The black letters refused to stay still. They danced and scrambled and reformed into riddles. "The... boy went to the studio to meet the photo-grapher," I read. (Not photographer.) "Which was the epi-thome...of..." (Not epitome.)

Then came the pause. And then the smirks. The shoulders shaking in silent laughter. The whispers weren't always quiet or kind in nature. Echoes stirred...

"What a dumbass." "Kid's a retard." "Jesus. Just stop reading."

Children can be cruel—but back then, they were unrestrained. There was no softening. No fear of consequence. No teachers intervening. Words like "retard" and "dumbass" flew through the air without shame. Laughter boomed across classrooms and made their way into locker rooms too. In the 70s and 80s, a boy's worth was tied to his toughness, and any deviation was grounds for open ridicule and quick dismissal.

And then there were my teeth. My goddamn teeth.

A dental curse passed down from someone I never met, made worse by childhood thumb-sucking and bad luck. My overbite was pronounced, the two front teeth bucked like a caricature. The names rolled in, again and again:

"Beaver Boy."
"Horse Face."
"Mr. Ed and Bucky."
"You could eat corn through a picket fence."

The worst one was simply: "Rake."

Admittedly, I was very slight and skinny as a middle schooler, but one kid said – "If you turned him upside down, he would make a great rake." Over time I became known to some as "Rake."

They said it all with such glee. They mimicked my voice, stuck out their jaws, turned my face into a playground joke. I began to hate mirrors. I learned to smile with my lips sealed. I stopped laughing out loud. And like many young teenagers, I then developed bad acne, and eventually I wanted to erase my face.

Mrs. Flanagan would sometimes give me a look—a soft, helpless gaze—the sad one, the kind adults give when they don't know what to do. Not compassion. Not really. Just the expression of someone watching a train wreck they can't stop. I hated that look more than the kid's laughter, mockery, and ridicule honestly. I didn't want her pity. I wanted invisibility.

After that, I began to vanish. In the hallways, I ducked behind taller kids, faked coughing fits, dropped pencils on purpose—anything to avoid being seen and worse, being called out. But the curse always came. My name always rose, seemingly somehow always in Mrs. Flangan's English class. Science class too. Science classes were particularly brutal for learning differentiated "disabled" children. The scientific names of insects, biology, and nature's organic function was way too much for my mind to comprehend, let alone try to sound out in front of my peers.

I didn't always know something was wrong. As a little boy, I just thought books were mean. They twisted and taunted. They weren't warm like cartoons or toys. They didn't laugh with me. They stared back coldly, daring me to understand. I would try—and fail. Again. And again.

My mother saw it first. The way I flinched at story time. The excuses I made. She saw the way I avoided bedtime stories, how I would make pleas to skip reading altogether. How I fidgeted, how my eyes danced across the page like they were looking for an escape hatch. My voice would falter on simple words, and I'd get mad—not at the book, but at myself.

My mother used to say, "Just keep plugging away." I know she meant no harm by this, I know she just wanted me to muscle through as if that were possible. But she did not know the irreversible harm and rage this caused within me.

The frustration. The rage, oh the rage when she said, "Just keep plugging away." It was her mindset that drove me crazy. Her thinking that persistence would equal brute-force through my neurological knots.

But it didn't help. It made it much worse, and she didn't understand that I was unraveling from the inside.

I remember one night in particular. I had a reading assignment. I stared at the page so long the letters blurred into a shadow. My mother sat beside me, trying to be gentle. "Just sound it out," she said. But the panic had already risen. My throat tightened. I slammed the book shut and told her violently, forcefully for her to get out of my room. With my face burning, giant sobs ripping from my chest like fire. That wasn't the first time. And it wouldn't be the last.

Eventually came the specialists. Gentle voices. Puzzles and tests. Clipboards and terms I didn't understand. Finally, words which professed my mental limitations and the cognitive conditions I possessed: mild dyslexia with significant reading comprehension issues – essentially, I had Learning Disabilities.

- Labels felt like life sentences.

Diagnosis:

1. Phonological Dyslexia (also called Dysphonetic)
- **Most common type.**
- Difficulty breaking words into phonemes (the sounds of speech).
- Trouble sounding out new or unfamiliar words.
- May guess words based on shape or context rather than decoding them.
- Example: Seeing the word "planet" and saying "place."

2. Surface Dyslexia (also called Dyseidetic)
- Struggles with recognizing whole words by sight (visual memory).

- Can sound out words phonetically but struggles with irregular words (like "colonel" or "island").
- Reads slowly and mechanically.
- Example: Misreading "yacht" as "yatched."

3. Rapid Naming Deficit Dyslexia

- Difficulty quickly naming letters, numbers, colors, or objects.
- Affects reading fluency and speed more than accuracy.
- Strong phonics skills may be present, but reading is still slow or effortful.

Secondary Diagnosis:

Significant reading comprehension issues refer to persistent and marked difficulty in understanding, processing, and retaining what is read, even when the individual can read words accurately and fluently. These issues go beyond simple reading struggles—they impair the ability to **derive meaning, make inferences, synthesize ideas, and connect information across texts.**

Core Characteristics:

1. **Difficulty Understanding Main Ideas**
   - Struggles to grasp the central theme or purpose of a passage.
   - May recall isolated facts but miss the "big picture."
2. **Poor Inference Skills**
   - Trouble reading between the lines or interpreting implied meaning.
   - Cannot easily connect information not stated explicitly.
3. **Weak Vocabulary**
   - Limited word knowledge hinders understanding.
   - Difficulty with figurative language, idioms, and nuanced phrasing.

4. **Working Memory Deficits**
   - Cannot hold and manipulate information long enough to integrate ideas across sentences or paragraphs.
   - May reread frequently and still forget what they just read.

5. **Trouble with Structure and Organization**
   - Fails to follow narrative or expository text structures.
   - Difficulty identifying cause and effect, sequencing, or comparing and contrasting ideas.

6. **Minimal Engagement or Mental Visualization**
   - Has trouble forming mental images while reading.
   - May not ask questions, make predictions, or reflect on the material.

Possible Underlying Causes:
- **Language Processing Disorders:** Weaknesses in receptive language (understanding) or expressive language (speaking).
- **Dyslexia or Reading-Based Learning Disabilities:** Especially when decoding takes so much effort that comprehension suffers.
- **ADHD or Attention Disorders:** Inability to maintain focus disrupts comprehension flow.
- **Low Background Knowledge:** Difficulty relating content to what they already know.
- **Emotional or Psychological Barriers:** Anxiety, trauma, or low self-esteem can block cognitive focus.

Signs in a Student or Reader:
- Might be able to read aloud fluently but doesn't understand what they read.
- Cannot summarize a passage or answer comprehension questions accurately.
- Often says, "I don't get it," or seems disengaged during reading activities.
- Needs constant rereading and prompting to understand text.

In Summary:

Significant reading comprehension issues are not just about reading words—they are about making meaning. When this skill is impaired, a person can feel as though they're looking at words through a foggy window: they can see the letters, but the message stays blurred. Recognizing and addressing the problem with empathy and strategy is key to unlocking deeper literacy and learning. Wow! Did you read that educational community? Recognizing and addressing the problem with empathy and strategy. Well, very little of these precious things called strategy or empathy was ever shown to me in my middle school and was not likely present in the public school system in the 1970s or early 1980s. Seems to me that the educators in my time were just as disabled, as I was, in helping me with my learning disabilities.

My father did help me though. Every Christmas, he would read, A Christmas Carol, by Charles Dickens. First published in 1843, the story tells the tale of Ebenezer Scrooge, a miserly old man who's transformed after being visited by the ghosts of Christmas Past, Christmas Present, and Christmas Yet to Come. More importantly it revealed the great character of Tiny Tim.

For those not familiar with A Christmas Carol by Dickens, Tiny Tim is a pivotal persona in this timeless Dickens classic. His full name is Timothy Cratchit, and he is the youngest son of Bob Cratchit, who works as a clerk for Ebenezer Scrooge. In Tiny Tim, I found a reflection of my own heart—a fragile, enduring kindred spirit. As he was a small boy, physically frail, and walked with the aid of a crutch.

Of course, his physical ailments and misalignment to the natural world, mirrored my reading comprehension struggles and mild dyslexia. He suffered from a serious, unnamed illness (likely something like rickets or tuberculosis, based on historical context). But despite his poor health, and the Cratchit family's poverty, he is remarkably kind, cheerful, and full of faith.

He is known for the famous line:
"God bless us, everyone!"

His importance in the story was not lost on me. Tiny Tim (Tiny) embodied innocence, goodness, and grace in a time where innocence, goodness and grace were sparse and times for his family were harsh and bleak. Though we never knew poverty or the weight of true hardship, I still identified with Tiny in my own way. To me, Tiny represents a pure-hearted boy, an innocent victim of social injustice—and children who suffer because of the negligence of the wealthy and powerful (in my case at the hands and tongues of the wicked and the cruel).

Tiny Tim showed me how even the weakest can have the strongest spirit. He became the driving catalyst for Scrooge's Transformation. When The Ghost of Christmas Yet to Come shows Scrooge that Tiny Tim will die if nothing changes, it deeply shakes him. And Tiny Tim's potential death becomes a turning point—a moral reckoning for Scrooge. It forces him to confront the human cost of his greed and indifference.

Because Scrooge changes his ways—becoming generous and compassionate—Tiny Tim survives. His recovery is not just a personal victory; it symbolizes hope, redemption, and the power of kindness to heal what greed neglects. To me Tiny Tim is the unlikely hero of A Christmas Carol by Dickens, and I yearned to be like him. A Christmas Carol gave me hope for humanity and hope for myself in the ways that Tiny could be saved by the transformation of others. I could not articulate this in my formative pre-teen years, but subconsciously the story somehow gave me great strength and optimism for a better future for myself.

In my time, my middle school responded poorly. I was pulled into side rooms, given books for children several years younger than myself, and treated like a pet project. Teachers called me distracted and lazy. Yet, I wasn't either. I was simply drowning, and no one could see the water.

The bullying only deepened. Kids weaponized everything. My voice. My face. My silence. The cafeteria was at times my own war zone. Every walk through the hallway, a trial. I stopped making eye contact. I kept to corners. I prayed, quietly, that the world would forget me.

I started hiding in the library, not because I loved books, but because I could pretend. I'd sit between the shelves, pretending to be busy. The library became a sanctuary—not for reading, but for disappearing.

Mrs. Velez, the librarian, was my first quiet protector. She never said much. But she left comics on the table for me, never asked questions, never forced me to read. Just left them there. A bridge. And one day, I crossed it.

I developed strategies and coping mechanisms. I memorized instead of reading. I became the self-deprecating clown. If I laughed at myself, maybe they wouldn't, or at least not as hard, or as harsh. But some days, the mask cracked. One teacher told me I was lazy. I smiled. I nodded. I went home and wept into my pillow like my body was splitting.

And then—a miracle. In eighth grade, it was like heaven sent an angel – Mrs. Langston.
She had long wavy blonde hair, tied in a loose bun. Sharp blue eyes, but not cold. She looked at me like I wasn't broken. More like I was a mystery worth unraveling. There was something sacred in her patience.

"I think you see the world differently," she said one day. "And that might be your gift."

She introduced me to horror greats: Edgar Allen Poe, Stephen King, and Mary Higgins Clark. Writers who described dark shadows and eerie metaphysical realities with such beauty it made my breath catch. These weren't stories. They were sanctuaries. Their pages didn't mock me— they haunted me. And in that haunting, I found refuge.

She taught me breathing techniques. She let me read at my own pace. One sentence at a time. One page at a time. She didn't try to fix me. She just stayed.

One day, she asked me to read aloud. Just her and me. I did. It wasn't perfect. But it was mine. And when she said, "You did it.", it felt like the first time someone saw me as whole, as unbroken.

She convinced my parents to consider a boarding school that specializes in students with learning differences. Back then they called them "disabilities," as if we were missing something instead of discovering a different language. What a cruel misnomer. No child is *learning disabled*. Only misunderstood, mismanaged, and mistaken as learning disabled.

Everything changed for the better, positively, when I arrived at Blue Ridge School in St. George, Virginia.

Blue Ridge's mission was simple and revolutionary for a boy like me: To help boys achieve their potential through personalized, structured, innovative learning practices in a college-preparatory, all-boarding community. I didn't understand the depth of that promise at first. But slowly, it became my oxygen. My rebirth.

At Blue Ridge, I was no longer a caricature. No longer the kid with the reading disorder and mental deficiency, the awkward smile, or dyslexic mind that refused to be quiet. I was a student. A learner. A boy with potential—not a problem to be fixed. Most of the other students, the other boys, were suffering in some way like me. The structure became a lifeline. There was predictability in the schedule, yes, but more importantly, there was belief. Teachers didn't look at me like I was broken—they looked at me like I was unfolding, blooming. My struggle was not a flaw; it was a feature. My way of learning wasn't strange or dysfunctional, it was unique and just mine.

For the first time in my life, I was taught how to learn in a way that honored who I was. Lessons were tailored. Expectations were firm but flexible. I didn't feel like I was dragging behind anymore—I was walking my own path, at my own pace, and that pace was respected.

Living among other boys in an all-boarding setting didn't erase the ache of the past, but it gave me the chance to rewire my idea of community. In the evenings, there were conversations. Laughter that didn't cut. Teachers who became mentors. They were friendships built not on hierarchy or cruelty, but on shared challenges, mutual growth, and late-night talks under star-flooded skies, sometimes even with campfires and tents. I once learned advanced geometry and algebra sitting in the snow—outside the classroom, at my desk—under the quiet guidance of my math teacher, Mr. Grant.

The immersive setting meant my support never ended at the classroom door. Faculty were present—not just as educators, but as steady presences. They noticed. They listened. They corrected gently. They praised sincerely. I wasn't just preparing for tests—I was preparing for life.

At Blue Ridge, I learned that independence didn't mean isolation. It meant responsibility. It meant trusting yourself to take the next step, even if your feet shook. It meant knowing you weren't walking alone.

The mission of the school wasn't a slogan. It was a covenant. A belief lived out through action. It turned survival into growth, and silence into song. It shaped me not only into a student capable of college—but into a man capable of compassion, introspection, and perseverance.

When I look back at those early years—the shame, the bullying, the self-erasure—I see a long, slow crucible. But I also see the teachers who pulled me out of the fire. I saw Mrs. Langston, and later, the entire team at Blue Ridge, who taught me that the only thing wrong with me was the belief that something was wrong at all.

The mission of Blue Ridge didn't just educate me. It liberated me. It gave me my mind back. My dignity. My voice. Thanks to Blue Ridge, I learned that difference isn't deficiency. It's design. And when a school leans into that truth, lives are not just changed—they're redeemed.

So now, when I speak to students, I don't just tell them about the boy who couldn't read, who had buck teeth and a broken voice. Who hid behind silence and pain, that he wasn't lazy, just unseen. And I tell them about a place that believed he could.

I show them the books I've written. I tell them about the horror of being misunderstood—and the miracle of finally being seen.

I wrote to silence them. I wrote to reclaim every word used against me. I wrote until pages stopped being enemies and became altars. I wrote until my voice grew roots.

I tell them about Mrs. Langston, Mr. Grant, and the entire Blue Ridge Team. And of my incredible transformative journey.

And I smile.
Fully. Brightly. Proudly.
Because some of us weren't born with straight lines.
We had to carve our own.

And now?
Now we write them, to.

BIO:

Jack Torrance is a critically acclaimed author of psychological thrillers and horror fiction that blend emotional intensity with chilling suspense. With an academic background in philosophy and psychology, Jack has spent over two decades crafting a singular brand of horror—one that doesn't merely frighten, but lingers, unravels, and possesses.

Known for turning trauma into art and obsession into poetry, Jack's narratives dive into the blurred boundaries between reality and madness. His prose is raw, lyrical, and deeply personal, confronting themes of grief, identity, mania, and the silence that festers beneath the surface of calm.

His breakout work, The Silent Canvas, and its haunting sequels have established him as a master of psychological dread, where love curdles into control, and memory becomes both a mirror and a weapon. In his collection When Horror Stares Back ~ Reflections of the Unseen, Jack explores the horrors that dwell not in monsters—but in the people we love, the voices we silence, and the truths we bury.

With a pen dipped in madness and shaped by memory, Jack Torrance writes to disturb, to disrupt, and to seduce readers into staring too long at what they fear most.

ROLLING WITH IT:
A Wheelchair Warrior's Unexpected Adventures
by Jeffrey VanDyke

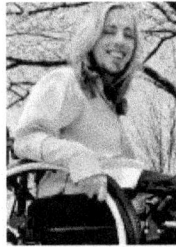

Chapter 1: My Grand (or Not-So-Grand) Entrance

Life, as they say, is a journey. Mine, however, started less like a scenic highway and more like a demolition derby. Forget the picturesque picket fence; my "gate" was more of a rusty, spike-covered monstrosity, guarded by fire-breathing dragons, swamp alligators, and possibly a grumpy troll toll collector. Welcome to the adventures of yours truly – helmets recommended, but not required (though, honestly, maybe invest in some good dental insurance).

Let's hit rewind on this highlight reel, shall we? My grand debut into this world was... well, let's just say it lacked any hint of glamour. I arrived about three months ahead of schedule, courtesy of a series of medical plot twists that would make a soap opera writer blush. And here's the kicker: my mom was offered a helicopter ride to the hospital for my dramatic entrance. A helicopter! Can you imagine the headlines? "Premature Prince Arrives by Chopper!" But alas—no Hollywood moment for me. She chose the classic ambulance route instead. (Cue disappointed groans from the imaginary audience.) I still say she robbed me of a red-carpet-worthy arrival.

But the drama didn't end there—oh no, that was just Act One. I eventually burst onto the scene (surprise!), but my breathing was... let's call it "enthusiastically problematic." Apparently, I stopped breathing multiple times, and the doctors—bless their concerned little hearts—gave me roughly two hours to live. Clearly, they didn't count on my tenacity. I channeled my inner Gloria Gaynor and, with all the strength a three-pound baby could muster, silently belted out, "I Will Survive!" Take that, grim prognosis!

Surviving the first few hours was just the beginning. What followed was a dizzying medley of pokes, prods, surgeries, and a feeding tube (I still joke that I could draw you a map of its route—big hit at kids' parties... not really). Complications? Oh, we had those in spades. It was practically a medical variety show. Looking back, I realize it was just the universe's way of preparing me for my future role: professional survivor.

Eventually, after what surely must've felt like an eternity of hospital life to my parents, I was finally cleared for takeoff—or at least the chance to go home. But something wasn't adding up—I wasn't hitting the usual developmental checkpoints. Crawling? Walking? Talking? I missed just about all of them, like someone skipping stones across a lake. The official diagnosis came around the age of two: Spastic Cerebral Palsy. And that, my friends, is when the real adventure began!

Chapter 2: My Wonky Hard Drive and the Great Jiggle

Ah, Spastic Diplegia Cerebral Palsy (SDCP). Catchy, isn't it? Sounds like a law firm or a particularly grumpy wizard. But let's be real, it's less "Harry Potter and the Spastic Diplegia" and more "My Life: A Comedy of Errors (and Involuntary Jerks)." For those unfamiliar, SDCP is basically my brain's way of saying, "Let's throw a party in your legs, and everyone's invited, especially Mr. Spasm and his pal, Mr. Stiffness!" Technically, it's a form of cerebral palsy that causes muscle stiffness and spasms, primarily in the legs and sometimes the arms. In my case, it also affects my speech. Think of it as my personal brand of interpretive dance—just without the artistic intention. It's all thanks to some slightly scrambled wiring in the ol' noggin. Apparently, I was so eager to join the party of life that I decided to RSVP way early. I practically catapulted myself out of the oven before the timer even dinged. Who needs a full nine months when you can launch into the world with nine seconds of unfiltered enthusiasm?

That early enthusiasm, combined with my signature jiggle (which puts Elvis' hip swivel to shame—seriously, I'm considering a lawsuit), means I navigate this magical landscape we call Earth from the comfort of my mobile steed: my wheelchair. It's a whole different world down here, let me tell you. I've become an expert in avoiding rogue shopping carts and mastering the art of the perfect wheelie. It's like my own personal Mario Kart adventure—just with fewer bananas and a lot more strategic parking.

Growing up with CP? Let's just say it was a character-building experience. I collected surgical scars like they were Pokémon cards—gotta catch 'em all! If you can name a medical procedure, chances are I've been there, done that, got the hospital gown. Especially during my mischievous years (which, let's be honest, are still ongoing). I was such a frequent flyer in the OR that I'm still mildly offended no one gave me a loyalty punch card. A personalized parking spot? A tiara? Something?

A lot of my early surgical highlights revolved around my ears—or more accurately, their refusal to function properly. The otolaryngologist (a.k.a. the ear, nose, and throat specialist—or ENT, because who has time for all that?) became my professional nemesis. I knew where those appointments were headed: more poking, more prodding, and the inevitable "Can you hear this?" Thirteen ear surgeries later—plus another twenty-something "odds and ends" procedures—I'd become a self-anointed pro. I could probably perform a tonsillectomy in my sleep... though I doubt anyone's lining up to let me try.

But my biggest medical showdown? That was with my spine. And at the tender age of four, it was time for our main event: a Selective Dorsal Rhizotomy (SDR). Think of it like a high-stakes game of Jenga—but your spine is the tower, and the goal is to remove just the right pieces without toppling the whole thing. No pressure. The mission? To reduce the spasticity—aka my muscles throwing a nonstop rave without my permission.

Thankfully, the surgery was a success! After a long hospital stay and some serious rehab, I didn't just gain function—I gained freedom. I could crawl more smoothly, dress myself (mostly), and use my arms in ways no one expected. And the real prize? I could finally pee like a boss. A true watershed moment, if you will.

While I'll always be a wheelchair user, there's no doubt those surgeries played a massive role in shaping my life. They were the foundation on which I built my empire of sarcasm and slightly off-kilter dance moves.

Chapter 3: School Daze (and My Mom's Superhero Cape)

Ah, school. The hallowed halls of learning, the joyous reunion of friends, the… abject terror of being separated from my mom for the first time. Okay, maybe I'm exaggerating a little. But let's be real, up until this point, my life had been a whirlwind tour of hospitals, doctors, and enough medical jargon to make a neurosurgeon's head spin. I'd become quite the connoisseur of sterile smells and the distinct squeak of hospital-grade linoleum. These experiences, while educational (I could probably diagnose a rare disease just by the sound of a cough), hadn't exactly prepared me for the social jungle of elementary school.

And speaking of jungles, my mom? She was basically Tarzan, swinging through bureaucratic vines and battling the beasts of "not-quite-accessible" architecture. Before I could even articulate a single coherent thought (my early vocabulary consisted mostly of "mama" and "more juice," neither of which are particularly helpful in an Individualized Education Plan (IEP) meeting), she was already a seasoned advocate. Forget capes, her superpower was unwavering determination. She wasn't just advocating for me; she was advocating for everyone. Think of her as a one-woman accessibility SWAT team, armed with a clipboard and an iron will.

Now, you might be thinking, "A wheelchair ramp? Lighter doors? That's what she was fighting for?" And yes, those were key battles. But they weren't just about me. They were about setting a precedent. It was about saying, "Hey, world, everyone deserves to be here. Everyone deserves to learn. And if that means you have to rearrange the furniture a little, then so be it." She wasn't just building ramps; she was building bridges. (Metaphorical bridges, of course. She left the actual construction to the professionals.)

My mom's advocacy wasn't just about getting me into school, it was about making sure I could navigate school. Think about it: a heavy door for someone in a wheelchair is like a locked gate. A missing ramp is like a moat. And let's not even talk about the horrors of a poorly placed fire alarm or worse a missing Evacuation Chair (a story for another chapter, trust me). My mom was preemptively striking against all these architectural evils.

So, there I was, this small human, armed with a backpack, which was probably twice my size, a Ninja Turtle figure or two in hand, and the legacy of my mom's fierce advocacy. School wasn't just a place of learning; it was a testing ground for her hard-won victories. And, as I soon discovered, a training ground for my own burgeoning advocacy skills. Because let's face it, when you've got a mom like mine, you learn that if you see something wrong, you don't just whisper about it – you shout it from the rooftops (or at least bring it up at the next IEP meeting). And that, my friends, is a lesson that would serve me well for years to come. Stay tuned for the next installment, where I learn the fine art of navigating cafeteria food and the even finer art of dealing with playground bullies.

Spoiler alert: my mom's influence extended far beyond the school's architectural design and served as the inspiration for the foundation that I still use today, when advocating for myself and others in our community.

Chapter 4: From Sick Days to Clicking Pixels (with Anxiety Detours)

My school years? Less High School Musical, more ER: Guest-Starring Yours Truly. Pneumonia, ear infections doing drum solos in my head, migraines that made sunshine public enemy number one, and random spasms—my body was basically a malfunctioning pinball machine.

Eventually, the constant medical drama subsided, freeing up some brain cells for actual schoolwork.

Enter Anxiety: the ultimate buzzkill.

Panic attacks became my unwelcome shadows. Thankfully, a supportive crew of therapists, cheerleading physical therapists, and some well-timed meds gradually turned down the volume on the internal screaming.

Despite feeling like a rolling WebMD entry, I somehow managed to pull off enough decent grades for an academic letter—and even snagged an arts scholarship to community college. But I was restless. Think: a caffeinated squirrel in a cage with no idea what direction to run.

Then came the call—the one that made my hands shake like a soda can after tumbling down a flight of stairs. It was about volunteering at Disability Network West Michigan.

Me? Volunteering? I felt about as qualified as a flip-flop in a snowstorm. But stepping into Disability Network was a revelation. Suddenly, I wasn't just "the wheelchair person." People saw me—really saw me. I soaked up skills like a dry sponge: résumé writing, interview ninja moves, public speaking. Programs like, "Job Club" and "My Choice, My Voice" showed me a world of possibilities I hadn't imagined.

And then, the shocker: I was awarded the Steven Silky Volunteer of the Year Award. Cue the happy internal screaming.

The even bigger shocker? They hired me—as their Graphic Design Specialist! Talk about a plot twist worthy of a daytime soap opera.

Now, I'm not just designing—I'm mentoring. I'm sharing my bumpy-but-ultimately-triumphant journey with others. Helping people find their own spark? Seriously rewarding.

Who knew one anxiety-ridden phone call would lead to this unexpectedly awesome adventure? Certainly not the past me, whose biggest daily goal was surviving without a full-blown panic attack.

Life, it turns out, has a quirky sense of humor.

Chapter 5: Rolling with Resilience (and a Dash of Sarcasm)

If anyone tells you navigating life is a cakewalk, they're probably selling something (or have a good baker). For me, as a wheelchair user with cerebral palsy, it's been less a leisurely stroll and more like an intricate tango – sometimes graceful, sometimes involving a rogue foot and a near-trip. Have there been days when the world felt like it was sitting squarely on my chest? Absolutely. Days when the challenges looked less like hurdles and more like Mount Everest in flip-flops. You bet. And the unsolicited opinions? Oh, the symphony of whispers and stares could rival a particularly dramatic opera.

But here's the thing I've learned: everyone's got their own version of Mount Everest in flip-flops. Maybe yours is a demanding boss, a tricky relationship, or just figuring out how to assemble flat-pack furniture without a meltdown. We all have our battles. Mine just happen to come with wheels and a side of wonky coordination.

However, amidst the noise and the occasional feeling of being an exhibit in a human zoo, something amazing happened: I found my voice. Not a booming, operatic voice (though sometimes I wish!), but a quiet, steady one that refused to be silenced by limitations or misconceptions. And honestly, it feels less like a desire to uplift and more like a personal mission – a responsibility I carry with a whole heart (and maybe a slightly clenched jaw when someone asks if I need "help" before even saying hello).

Because here's the truth, my friends: this wheelchair? It's not my kryptonite. It's more like my Batmobile. It gets me where I need to go, allowing me to soak in all the glorious, messy, hilarious beauty this world has to offer. From belly laughs with friends that make my abs ache (the good kind!) to those quiet moments of staring at a sunset and feeling a profound sense of peace, every experience is a thread in the tapestry of my life. And I'm determined to weave a vibrant, positive pattern.

Chapter 6: When My Superhero Took Off Her Cape (Too Soon)

Just as my self-discovery journey was starting to hit its stride—picture an awkward baby giraffe learning to walk, but with more existential pondering—life threw a curveball harder than a Nolan Ryan fastball.
My mom—my original gangster of advocacy, the woman who could charm a grumpy badger into signing an accessibility petition—was suddenly diagnosed with Stage 4 lung cancer. It felt like a cosmic prank. A bad joke with zero punchline.
For the next 18 months, she fought like a warrior queen going head-to-head with a particularly persistent dragon (that dragon being cancer—and trust me, it's the nastiest kind). There were surgeries, treatments, enough medical appointments to rack up frequent flyer miles in the oncology ward—all while the world wrestled with the chaos of the COVID pandemic.

Ultimately, despite her incredible strength and an army of medical professionals, my mom laid down her metaphorical sword of advocacy. Losing her wasn't just heartbreaking; it felt like a fundamental shift in the universe. She was my North Star—the one who taught me how to bounce back from life's inevitable gut-punches and the unfiltered, no-holds-barred power of love.

Her advocacy wasn't a phase—it was her superpower. And now, it's up to me: the slightly less coordinated but equally determined next-gen advocate, to pick up that sword. It's a daunting task—like trying to follow Beyoncé's choreography after watching a single YouTube tutorial. But I owe it to her to keep the mission going—with the same fire in my belly, the same unwavering dignity, and the same fierce grace she lived by every single day.

So, here's to you, Mom.

Your cape may be hung up, but your legacy? That's just getting started. And trust me—I plan on making some noise. You taught me well. Oh—and if you were expecting a quiet, dramatic exit? Picture this: Me, attempting a slow-motion wheelie while tossing metaphorical glitter. Graceful? Debatable. Memorable? Absolutely.

Chapter 7: The Grand Finale (Confetti Included)

The big takeaway I hope you're rolling away with is this: disability isn't the villain in life's story—it's more like an unexpected detour with some surprisingly scenic views. It's just another facet of the wonderfully weird diamond that is humanity. Some of us sparkle in one way, some in another. I just happen to come with built-in seating and a unique perspective on curb heights. It's all good.

My mission in life isn't about conquering the world, one inaccessible ramp at a time (though that would be a satisfying side quest). It's about spreading love and hope with the enthusiasm of a toddler holding a confetti cannon. I want to be remembered as the guy who could find the funny bone in a pile of adversity—who looked for the silver lining, even when it was playing hide-and-seek behind a thundercloud.

As the insightful Helen Keller once said:
"Optimism is the faith that leads to achievement. Nothing can be done without hope and confidence."

And that's my parting thought for you, dear reader.
Wherever you are in your own epic tale—whether you're just turning the first page or you're a seasoned narrator—keep writing. Life throws plot twists that would make M. Night Shyamalan jealous, but there's always room for a new chapter full of possibility.

So: embrace your quirks. Chase your dreams (even the slightly far-fetched ones). And believe—fiercely—in your own strength.

Let my journey, with all its bumps and triumphs, be a gentle nudge to take that next step, no matter how small. You've got this. Seriously.
Now go out there and shine your unique light. The world needs it.
And from my corner of Muskegon, Michigan, consider this your standing ovation.

You're amazing. Now, roll on.

BIO:

Born with cerebral palsy and a lifelong wheelchair user, **Jeffrey VanDyke** has woven his unique perspective into a vibrant tapestry of artistic expression and dedicated advocacy. As both a talented author and a published children's book illustrator, his creativity knows no bounds. Beyond his art, Jeffrey actively engages as an adaptive athlete and a passionate disability advocate. He is driven by a profound commitment to fostering inclusivity and understanding, hoping to leave a legacy of a more accessible and representative world for all. Jeffrey's work serves as an inspiration, encouraging others
to celebrate their individuality.

www.facebook.com/jeffrey.vandyke
www.linkedin.com/in/jeff-vandyke

THE REIGN *AFTER THE RADIANCE*

Born at the Edge of Dawn
by Jenny L. Ford

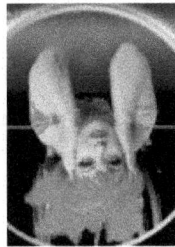

"When the light slipped from my skin, I learned to become the sun myself."

Every pore of my being was relaxed, as though time itself had paused to savor the stillness. Just me and the water. A weightless sense of bliss dissolved all of my cares, leaving me in a deep, tranquil calm, in the front yard, in a large pool, shaded by the new screened-in tent cover. I was a child of the South, though now, in my late twenties. I loved the Texas sun, its rays soothed me, gifting me a saffron-robed tan and rosy cheeks. Hawaiian Tropic Coconut Oil skimmed the surface of the water, and I was reading on my floaty. How I had missed this!

Yet, I had learned to tread carefully, like Eos herself bound to the fleeting beauty of the dawn, knowing that to linger too long might invite a cruel twist of fate. Like her, I had reveled in the sun's warm embrace, only to find myself cursed by its power. I had been drained, and sun exposure had begun to make me ill. Painful rashes, those strange and excruciating blisters, had claimed me as their unwilling victim. Today, though, was different. The shade promised safety. My little piece of perfection. My brief respite.

But just as the goddess of the dawn is forever separated from the full radiance of day, so too would my last rendezvous with the sun outside the dawn hours end. In the next moments, everything would change.

There was no slope. No warning. One moment, bliss. The next, **excruciating pain.** Instantly. It felt like a billion fire ants had bitten me all at once. No, bitten and burrowed. A billion wasps stung at the same time, like nature had declared war on my skin. Nausea hit me like a wave, and I vomited. Then everything locked. My body froze in place. **Paralyzed by pain.**

But eventually, movement returned. Barely. I leapt from the pool, stumbled inside, and dove into the shower, thinking cold water would soothe it. Instead, it felt like acid ran down my spine. I screamed. Tears, snot, sweat. Everything poured out of me in waves. I was a waterfall of panic and fire. Somewhere, through the static of pain, I knew **I was losing my mind.** One millisecond at a time.

I grabbed the phone and called the EMS station where my wife was on duty. She answered, but she didn't understand. How could she? Instead of coming to get me, she suggested I stop by her grandmother's house to grab some Silvadene cream. She thought it was just a sunburn. I didn't even put on clothes. Still in my swimsuit, I got in the car. And I drove. **Forty-five minutes round trip.**

Screaming & Crying **EVERY SINGLE SYLLABLE** of "The Sound of Madness" album by Shinedown. The irony was not lost on me. That is a story for another day.

When I arrived at the station, we applied the Silvadene. The moment it touched my skin, it was like pouring salt on open wounds, the stings, the bites, the fire, **the acid.** I collapsed.
Lost consciousness.

Diagnosis: Acute Cutaneous Lupus Erythematosus.
A severe photosensitivity reaction. The most intense form—Bullous Lupus Erythematosus.

That day, the sun betrayed me. And I have avoided it like the plague ever since. Living in Texas, this has been an especially cruel paradox. The sun, once my sacred place of peace, became a silent predator. And there has been much misery. Much misunderstanding. Much unlearning. I had to forge a new kind of relationship between my body and the heat. Because it's not just the rays. It's the **swelter**, the suffocation. The heat itself became its own kind of violence.

In the **Chapters of Defiance**, I endured many days that mirrored that first horrific one. Days where I pushed through, tried to "shake it off," pretended that willpower could outrun biology. And then came the **Chapters of Acceptance,** Longer, slower, quieter. Days of trying to navigate life fully covered, head to toe, in 115-degree heat. Still a mother. Still a wife. Still expected to show up for work, for people, for dreams. And all of it while sick. Uninsured.

I couldn't be added to my wife's insurance. Because at the time, LGBTQ+ marriages weren't recognized, and insurance companies chose not to provide coverage. The system had its own gatekeepers. Then there was the grief. Not just of health, but of friendships that faded, relationships that couldn't hold this version of me, foods my body once loved but now violently rejected, routines, outings, even clothes. So many tiny deaths. But somewhere after rage, after despair, after bargaining, came stillness. Then, the truth. Then, boundaries. Then, self-value. Then, **worthiness**. And eventually **Celebration.**

The celebration of saying yes. The power of saying no. The clarity of recognizing that the sun can be felt and honored in ways beyond standing beneath it. It lives now in my citrus tea. In the laughter of my child. In golden light streaming through the curtains. In lemon-colored blankets. In the way my skin glows from within, no longer needing to prove anything to the sky.

Before I move forward, before we drift too far from that poolside epiphany and into the long walk that followed, there are things I must say.

As a child, I was already living with an invisible constellation of conditions. Diagnosed early with **migraines**, **autism**, and **ADHD**, my nervous system was always wired differently. Even then, the quiet signals of **lupus** had begun to whisper unnoticed, unconnected, unexplained, their first murmurings traced back to when I was just 2.

But the full diagnosis? It would take **decades**. By the time they gave it a name, I had already survived a thousand unnamed battles. Just six months before that sunlit trauma, I had finally been diagnosed with **fibromyalgia** after **over a decade** of chronic, debilitating symptoms. And it came at a cost.

That diagnosis marked the loss of my career. Not a job. A calling. One, I had **broken family chains** to achieve. Because I had done the impossible. I had once been a single mother with no vehicle, no government assistance, and a toddler on my hip, and still, I built something for us. I rose. I became. Only to watch it all unravel because my body began rewriting its own code.

Please **do not lose me here.** Do not let the heaviness of this part cause you to shut the book. This is a story about **the unsugarcoated truth**. About what a diagnosis actually looks like. About the ripple effects that medicine doesn't always document, the loss of identity, the breakdown of relationships, The dreams you bury quietly because no one claps for pacing yourself.
Being more than your diagnoses doesn't mean skipping over it. It means **naming the full truth**: the stumbling, the spirals, the false recoveries that have you thinking, "Maybe I'm better," only to be met again with pain that says, "NO" with a tear of its own because *YOU* **DO NOT UNDERSTAND.**

And I can't sleep at night as an author

If I don't tell that truth.

Because I know, I know, someone out there is reading this from a couch they haven't left in days. Wondering if they're the only ones. If the weight they carry is just theirs. If their symptoms are too strange, too specific, too shameful to speak aloud. This chapter—this entire book—is for them.

Yes, there will be more diagnoses. More names. More complications. But there will also be the ways I lived with them. Not despite them. **With them.** There will be the tools, the holistic approaches, the mindfulness practices, the western prescriptions, the eastern traditions, the spiritual, the sacred, the skeptical, and the science.

Because over thirty years of navigating evolving autoimmune conditions has taught me this: There is no one path through. There is only the **honest path**. And I'm still walking it. Just 3 days ago, I was diagnosed with my 8th Autoimmune Disease.

Before marriage was legal, before my doctor even considered that the symptoms I carried might be lupus, before I had access to insurance for anything outside of emergency situations, my first love died. And I became a widow. Not in title.

But in truth.

The next **nine years** would find me surviving through sheer willpower. ER visits instead of preventive care. Marijuana and cigarettes for pain relief. Yoga, when I could stretch. Meditation when I could sit still. Exercised until I collapsed. Diet until my body rejected even the healthiest foods. Prayer. So much prayer. A **bipolar** journey of ups, downs, and crashing waves wrapped in **CPTSD and anxiety**, all folded into the quiet chaos of an undocumented war within my body.

Three years into a second marriage. Still no insurance. Still no ability to work. Then, one morning after eating, Pain deep and cruel settled in my gut. A rock that refused to pass. It stayed for days. Then came a flood of symptoms: vomiting, weight loss, weakness. I lost the ability to eat my carefully chosen, clean foods. Even sipping water felt like punishment. And so began the next evolution of survival: **Pedialyte in wine glasses** to keep my spirit from shattering. **Baby**

food asnourishment, swallowed with tears. I did this for **five years**.

While a hole grew in my stomach, spilling out not just food, but parts of who I had been.

Eventually, the diagnosis came: **Ulcerative Colitis. Crohn's Disease.** Words that spelled out what my life had become: fragmented, inflamed, and misunderstood.

The day I "landed" in a wheelchair, I was driven to my now adult son's home. He carried me up the stairs, cradled my weight in silence, and laid me gently on his couch. And without a word spoken, that was the day I became **a new divorcée for the second time.** There was no need for a ceremony. It was clear. That chapter had ended.
And there…**there**… the tide turned.

Within weeks of that ending, I was reborn into something new. I moved into my twin brother's home in a new state, with **new health laws**, **different access**, and, as it turns out, a very different kind of mercy. Within **days** of arriving, I was in the emergency room. Unlike the past, this time I wasn't dismissed. I was **approved for surgery** on the spot. My **gallbladder was removed**, and other urgent repairs were made.

Very quickly, almost impossibly so, I met and married the **great love of my life.** And for the **first time in my life**, I gained **health insurance**. **Real** healthcare.

A right that had always been treated as a privilege. Now, finally, mine. A rapid-response team of specialists was assembled like clockwork, each one tackling a part of the whole I'd been experiencing shatter, alone.

First: A **gastric specialist** who brought in a **weight specialist** to save the mere **15%** of my stomach I had left. They performed a reconstructive surgery, similar to a **gastric sleeve**, designed not for weight loss, but for survival. Then came four **life-altering medications**.

A family practitioner who listened, really listened, and prescribed three more meds with the precision of someone who believed I deserved to be well.

A **rheumatologist**, my lifeline, who handed me three more tools in the form of prescriptions, each one easing the inflammatory fires within me.
A **cardiologist**—two medications.
A **hematologist**—two more.
The list grew, and so did my ability to **function**.
To **trust**.
To **breathe**.

I was no longer cobbling together wellness from scraps. I was finally given a team, a plan, a second chance at being alive with resonance.
I have not flailed it. No. I have not flailed in this life.
Yes, I've watched my disease processes evolve like wild tides, pulling new diagnoses from the depths. Yes, I've had more surgeries. Yes, the daily challenges are many. Some visible. Most invisible. All real. But I have also **thrived**.

I have lived as death, and I have lived as healing. And somehow, somehow, healing became almost **effortless**, not because it was easy, but because I stopped fighting myself. I began to flow with the truth of my body.

In the midst of it all, I have acquired **several certifications**. I have **helped others** launch their dreams I have launched my **own business**, one rooted in authenticity, service and sacred vision. I have pursued the shimmer of possibility with open arms, and the **limitless universe** has whispered back, "Yes."

I have returned again and again to the quiet rituals that restore me: **routines**, **creative work**, **collaboration**, **art**, **beauty**, and **Co-creation**. I have relearned the **miracle of sleep** even if it comes at odd hours. And when it doesn't come, I write. I dream while wide awake. Most of this chapter you're reading? It was written by hand in the half-light. Scrawled in a **bedside notepad**, at 2:00 a.m., when my body feels unsteady but my spirit is clear.

I write through the ache. I write through the tremor. I write because the dream refuses to die. And because the dreamer still lives here, there are mornings now not many, but some where the sun peeks through the window, and I do not shrink. I do not run from the light. I watch it. I feel it from a distance. I welcome its presence like an old teacher, one who once burned me but who now glows just enough to remind me that I still exist.

The sun and I...we are no longer adversaries. We are **witnesses** to each other. I have learned to revere it in shadows, in filtered light, in warm-toned art, in heatless flame. Because I have become my own sun.

This is what no one tells you about chronic illness, about invisible disabilities, about autoimmune shapeshifting and life-altering diagnoses: **It's not linear.** It's not tidy. It's not about "getting better." It's about becoming. Again. And again. And again.

Healing, for me, did not come wrapped in a single pill or path. It came in fragments in medicine bottles and essential oils, in tear-soaked pillows and burning sage, in yoga mats and wheelchairs, in sleepless nights and 2 a.m. journal pages, in fierce boundaries and soft forgiveness, in saying "no," and in finally whispering "yes" to the parts of me I had long rejected. It came when I stopped trying to go back to who I was, and started letting who I was becoming…lead me forward.

This chapter is not just a testimony of survival. It is a map. For anyone who has ever sat in a fluorescent-lit waiting room, staring at a clipboard full of boxes that could never hold your whole story. For anyone who's ever been dismissed, misdiagnosed, underestimated, left behind by a system that was never built to understand bodies like ours.

This chapter is not to inspire pity. It is not to wrap hardship in a bow. It is not to pretend that transformation makes the pain worth it. It is to say: **You are not alone.** And you are not broken. And you are not a burden. You are not "too sensitive." You are a tuning fork for a world that no longer listens. You are a lighthouse in a storm that never gave you a warning. You are a phoenix still in the ash, **and you still count.**

There are days I still cry in the shower. There are days I still grieve what I cannot do. There are days the pain folds me in half. But I have also laughed so hard my scars shook. I have created art that made people weep. I have held space for others the way no one once did for me.
I have chosen softness. I have built altars. I have kissed the palms of the ones I love and told them, "This is sacred." And I have told myself the same thing, over and over and over: **"This life is still sacred."**

So now, when I wake up at the edge of dawn, my pen in hand, my body uncertain, my dreams half-sketched on crumpled paper, I remind myself: After the radiance, the reign.

When the light slipped from my skin, I didn't disappear. I became. Not the sun's subject, but its mirror. It's keeper. It's echo. It's flame. This is not the end. This is not the peak. This is the breath before the next rise. I am not healed. I am not healing. But I am not done. I am **becoming**. Born at the edge of dawn and still glowing.

The first time I experienced remission, I jumped up and down on the inside. I told everyone that I was "healed by the blood of Jesus!" (Please do feel free to hear that in an exaggerated, slightly jaded, southern drawl.) That was the extreme difference. I woke up and it was almost as if I hadn't been fighting for my life for years. This lasted for 3 days.

Then, I fell victim to my own fear, to the Southern Baptist indoctrination that had shaped so much of my early life. This religion of my youth whispered that sickness was a consequence. That somewhere, somehow, I had let the devil in.

And now, with this momentary relief stripped from my body, I believed I had a chance to cut out the root of his entrance. To purify. To cleanse. To repent.

I went to war against myself. I fasted, I wept, I begged God to make it permanent. I blamed myself for every flare-up that came after. I believed…truly…that if I just did enough spiritual work, if I just uncovered and confessed enough sins, I could stop being a person who was ill.

No one told me, not once, what remission was. That I could experience it. That it was a normal part of a permanent disease. No one told me the rhythm of it, that wellness could return for a time and still be part of the illness. No one told me I didn't need to earn my healing or blame myself when the cycle returned.

So instead of peace, I suffered. Greatly. Not from the disease alone, but from the self-persecution I piled on top of it. Because when you're taught to believe you're the reason for your suffering, every moment of relief becomes a test:

Are you good enough to keep it? Holy enough to deserve it? Worthy enough to stay well?

And that kind of thinking? It scars deeper than the illness. Eventually, painfully, I began to understand something I now hold sacred: even disease longs to be witnessed. It needs what we all need, to be seen, heard, understood. To not be cast out as punishment, but held as a messenger. As a part of the whole, not a sign of failure. When I finally stopped exorcising my body like it was evil, I began to hear what it was really trying to say.

Not, "You are wrong."

But:

"You are overwhelmed."

"You are inflamed."

"You are carrying too much."

"You need rest, not repentance."

That was when the tide turned again. Not because I was healed, but because I stopped equating healing with righteousness. Here is the absolute reality: From the moment of birth, our bodies begin to deteriorate, ultimately leading to death through the passage of time and various medical conditions. But that is not a reason to fear. It is a reason to honor.

To LIVE

My diagnoses have taught me so many deeper meanings about life. What I rejoice in the most is not the myth of purpose, but the liberation from the plague of dogma that told me purpose must be earned through pain. I do not believe we are here to suffer into significance. Purpose, in the old paradigm, was a carrot dangled in front of us to keep us striving, grinding, proving. But I have come to understand: we are here to remember.

To BE.

Resonance, not purpose, is what I follow now. And resonance lives in moments, not mandates. It is not a divine task list. It is not assigned by a system. It is a vibration felt in truth, in awe, in connection. My diagnoses activated that remembrance within me. That I am not here to earn love. That I am not broken. That being is enough. That rest is not lazy. That softness is not weakness. That my value was never tethered to performance. When I surrendered to this truth, I found that my breath deepened.

My boundaries sharpened. My joy expanded.

And the sun? The same sun that once betrayed me became, once again, a symbol of illumination. Not for punishment.

Now I know: Even when I am aching. Even when I am grieving. Even when I am unsure of what tomorrow will ask of me, I am glowing. Not because I have "overcome," But because I have undergone.

I have passed through fire, through waters that tried to drown me, through systems that tried to silence me. And I emerged not untouched, but unchained.

If you are reading this and you are somewhere in your own descent, please know: This is not your ending. You don't need to become radiant by someone else's definition. You don't need to return to the version of you who existed before the diagnosis, before the rupture, before the unraveling.

You are allowed to be someone new. Someone wiser. Someone softer. Someone more tuned in to life's quiet miracles. Someone who holds grief and joy in the same breath.

Because this is what time has taught me: There is no straight line. There is no clean before-and-after. There is only the sacred middle where you breathe through the ache, dance through the limits, and learn to love the life that fits your form, not the one others expected you to squeeze into. And in that space? You create. You redefine. You reign.

Not the reign of conquest but the reign of inner authority. Of choosing to live aligned with your own rhythm. A radiant return to the self. I no longer chase "normal." Normal never fit me anyway. What I chase now, if you can call it chasing, is resonance. Connection. Peace that does not rely on productivity. Beauty that isn't skin-deep but soul-deep. A kind of strength that isn't measured by miles walked, but by the courage to stay soft in a world that expects you to harden.

I've learned that living your best life sometimes means crying in a locked bathroom then emerging with mascara streaks and still choosing to show up. It means canceling plans. It means honoring fatigue. It means choosing joy without needing permission. It means not apologizing for your pain and not downplaying your progress.

It means rewriting what it means to thrive. So if you, too, were born at the edge of something: A diagnosis, a disaster, a shift you never saw coming...

Know this:

There is life after the fall. And not just survival. There is radiance. There is reign. There is the reclamation of your own rhythm. So find your shade tree. Pour your Pedialyte into a wine glass if you must. Write your truth at 2:00 a.m. Let your body speak its language, and learn to answer with compassion instead of contempt.

This life may not look like the one you planned. But it can still be yours. Still rich. Still tender. Still holy, born at the edge of dawn and still glowing.

BIO:

Jenlyn Ford is a #1 international best-selling co-author, globally recognized disability advocate, disability leader, brand stylist, speaker, and founder of Uniqua New Beauty Norm LLC, where rebellion becomes ritual and authenticity is crowned. A multi-dimensional storyteller, she weaves together mythology, neuroscience, resilience, and avant-garde artistry to breathe life into narratives that defy labels and ignite transformation.

Her words pulse through acclaimed anthologies including Beyond Boundaries: Thriving in Life's Grey Zone (The Seasoning), The Legacy Chronicles: A Message to My Family (Forged in Breath), A People First Professional Network Platform (The Trilogy: Book One) (The Universe is Mental), and Phoenix of Resilience Rising from Adversity (I Will Be Your Angel). Each chapter disrupts the myth of limitation, inviting readers to see that need, frailty, and divergence are not weaknesses; they are the architecture of sovereignty.

Diagnosed with SLE Lupus, Crohn's disease, Rheumatoid Arthritis, Fibromyalgia, Parkinson's +, Jenlyn embodies the truth that it is not despite her challenges, she thrives, but because of the powerful systems they forged. As a cinematic brand stylist, audacious neurodivergent leader, and fierce disability advocate, she helps multi-passionate creators transform their lived experiences into breathing brands and revolutionary legacies.

In We Choose to Be More Than Our Diagnoses, Jenlyn stands boldly in the light: her diagnoses did not chain her, they crowned her. Through conscious systems, sacred breath, and fierce remembrance, she reminds us: when the light slips from our skin, we are meant to become the sun ourselves.

SENTENCED TO THE ELECTRIC CHAIR:
This Wasn't The Plan, But Here We Are
by Jerry Ryan

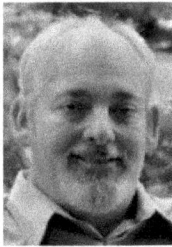

My life changed on an Easter Sunday morning.

My sons asked if we could go for a ride in the car. We hadn't gotten to do much riding in it the day before when we bought it at the used car dealership.

We lived in a subdivision of Albuquerque that bordered the desert. Within a mile of our house, there was a road being put in for a new subdivision. The area was closed off to traffic but that only took a little maneuvering around the gate to get onto the road. We drove out about a mile, turned around, and started to come back.

The sun was beautiful and sparkled on the Sandia Mountains as we came down a long straight stretch of road. You couldn't have asked for a better day or better driving conditions.

Bang! Suddenly, the right rear tire shredded like a retread and wrapped around the rear axle. The car locked up and started spinning to the left. It slid into the desert and struck a small rise in the sand, catapulting it fifteen feet into the air. The car flipped upside down and landed on the driver's side roof, crushing it down to the door. It then flipped onto its wheels and came to a sudden stop.

I couldn't move and I couldn't breathe. I looked over to my right and saw my 13-year-old son, Daniel. He was okay; just banged up. I tried to look in the back seat to check on my 15-year-old son David, but I couldn't turn my head. I couldn't see or hear him. That was because he had been thrown from the vehicle and landed about 50 feet away on his hands and knees. When he came running up to my window, he only had a scar on his shin from going through the window during the accident.

Daniel ran to call for help while David got my seatbelt off. Because of my years in the medical field, I knew that I had broken my neck. But I could not tell my kids that. David followed my directions to get me safely out of the vehicle because it was starting to smoke, and we were worried that it would catch fire.

Life works in an amazing way. Even though we were on a closed road on Easter Sunday morning in 1994, the first person that appeared on the scene was a trauma nurse with a cell phone. She was riding her bike on the closed road that morning. She took over, put my son at ease, and called for the ambulances. I was taken to the University of New Mexico. My sons were taken to a different hospital across town. I can't begin to imagine the stress that my wife Marcy felt that day.

Because of the intense physical damage, I have little memory of the accident or the three months following it. It turns out that I was right about breaking my neck but that was only the tip of the iceberg of injuries that I had.

I had pulverized my seventh vertebrae in my neck, twisted my spinal cord into a tight "S" at that point, broke my left collarbone, shattered my left shoulder blade into five pieces, broken all the ribs on my left side, punctured my left lung, dislocated my left arm, and wiped out both frontal lobes of my brain.

One of the doctors told me afterward that they only see an injury like mine once every four or five years and that's during an autopsy. Over a year later, a doctor told me that according to my brain scans, I should be drooling and unable to make complete sentences. It's nice to have proved them both wrong.

My injuries were so bad that within the first 15 minutes of me being in the emergency room, the doctors took my wife to a separate room and asked her to sign a "Do Not Resuscitate" order. She refused and told them to get back there and do their jobs. I will forever owe my life to her decision that day.

I spent three months in and out of reality, sometimes being present in the moment and other times living in a world of drug- and fever-induced hallucinations.

I remember repeating one word in my mind while I was in the ICU. It meant the difference between life and death. The word was BREATHE.

When I actually "awoke," I was in a rehabilitation hospital and the pain was incredible! I was bound up in a halo-like device that was strapped to my chest and screwed into my head.

When I looked down at my body, the muscles that I had spent years developing were gone. I couldn't move anything but my eyes and my right arm. But I could only get my right hand to my mouth twice before it was too hard to move. None of my fingers could move so I couldn't even hold a spoon or fork to feed myself.

To make things even more stressful, I had tubes in both my nostrils and other tubes coming out of various places in my body. I avoided looking in the mirror and I could see the fear in my sons' eyes when they came to visit.

As I became more alert to what was going on, I learned that my family support had kicked in the day after the accident. Two of my younger brothers came down on the first flight, went directly to the crash site, and took pictures of the remnants of tire and the skid marks leading to the desert.

My parents loaded up their motor home and drove from Portland to Albuquerque. They stayed parked in the hospital parking lot for almost two months. My family is definitely one of the things that saved my life.

I spent three months in the rehab hospital getting back my strength and stamina so I could go home. It involved a lot of physical therapy, counseling, and exposure to my new world of paralysis in a power wheelchair.

My body was a prison and I was sentenced to an electric chair.

There is a lot of stress involved in something as life changing as losing the ability to move your body. Suddenly, everything in life requires help from somebody else. Everything includes day-to-day routines that we all take for granted like turning in bed, getting dressed, getting up in the morning, eating meals, bathing, and even using the bathroom.

I was incredibly lucky to have had great staff while in the rehabilitation unit. One of the people who help me keep my mind in the right place was the night shift nurse, Art.

We would have "midnight talks." He was preparing me for what my life would be like after I got back into the real world. Art would tell me, "Don't be like Mr. Smith in room 108. All he does is feel sad and cry all the time." He would continue, "And don't be like Mr. Taylor in room 115. All he does is yell at people and throw things any time someone tries to help him."

I could certainly understand why nobody would want to be constantly sad or angry, but Art was making a different point. "The last thing you want to do is to alienate the people that you will need for the rest of your life," he said.

I took what he said to heart and began thanking every staff person, friend, and family member.

I went on my first interaction with the public when the recreational therapist took several of us on an outing to the local mall. I felt like all eyes were on me as I rolled through the mall that I had walked through many times before. I thought that I should be marking the moment with a reward, so I went into one of the stores to purchase earrings.

After managing to find a pair that I liked, I approached the checkout stand with earrings in my left hand and a $20 bill in my right. I sat and watched as a customer walked up from my left and was waited on.

Another approached from my right and was waited on. I wondered why I wasn't being waited on.

I finally asked the clerk, "Am I just too short?" Using humor seemed to get the clerk's attention without causing embarrassment. Little did I know that I would be needing to use this humor over and over again in public situations in the future.

There were daily struggles with trying to get movement back in my body. Moving my arms was the focus and every movement caused a spike in the burning and tingling pain. Intense pain came from all movements of my body and with all physical contact.

For a while, I was stuck in the "Why Me?" mindset. A friend of mine was visiting and asked me "What if it's not about you? What if it's about everybody you meet for the rest of your life?" Those questions were a wakeup call that still guides my life.

My family continued to be a great source of support. My wife, my sons, my parents, and my in-laws were reminders that I was not alone. They gave me a reason to keep going despite the agonizing pain.

At one point, my father was alone with me in the rehab hospital. He began crying and told me that this wasn't what he thought my future would be. I promised him that if I had to be a quadriplegic, I'd be the best one ever.

Words have power. I had no idea how powerful the words of that promise would be.

Another one of the things that gave me strength in the rehab unit was the continuous stream of visitors that were my hearing aid clients. You never really know how much you impact a person's life.

That was made clear to me when some of my clients would drive for over an hour to come and visit me for 15 or 20 minutes. They would tell me how important what I had done for them was and what a change it had made in their lives with their families.

But not everyone that visits the rehab unit is a good person. One night, we were sitting outside my room on the patio when I began to have a problem. We rushed back into the room and called the medical staff. It all took less than five minutes and then my wife realized that she had left her purse sitting by the chair on the patio. Stepping outside the door, she looked and saw that it was gone.

Marcy returned the next day to have lunch with me. She had the extra keys to the Jeep so she could drive it home. After having a stunning lunch of hospital food, she left to go home. Within five minutes, she returned with a stunned look on her face. The people who had stolen her purse the night before had returned to steal her Jeep out of the parking lot at lunch time. It was there when she arrived, but it was gone when she went to leave. The only thing that we could do was look at each other and bust out laughing. What else could happen?

To add to the stress that I was already dealing with because of the quadriplegia, my family and I engaged in a lawsuit against the car dealership, their inspection service, and the tire manufacturer.

After months of meetings and a trial which made the front page of the Albuquerque newspaper, the car dealership and their inspection service chose to settle out of court. The tire manufacturer was a billion-dollar corporation and had more than enough money to use the legal system to their benefit. However, the out-of-court settlements provided us with an ongoing safety net.

After getting out of the hospital, we moved back to Portland. Even though we had moved back to a place that had more resources and support from my family, life continued to throw curveballs. But this wasn't my first time at bat in life, so I knew the rules of the game and how to use them.

Change was not a new thing for me. It started when I was a kid.

My father's federal job meant we moved often. I attended eleven different schools in twelve years. Each year brought the stress of being the new kid again.

The bullying started in second grade, in what should have been a safe place – the boys' bathroom. That space became a war zone for years.

By high school, I turned to alcohol and drugs to cope.
But things began to shift when I joined a judo class at the YMCA. It wasn't just about learning to defend myself. Martial arts gave me a sense of focus and strength.

I got a weightlifting set and started reading about yoga and meditation. For the first time, I found tools that helped me take charge of my life.

In college, I worked full-time while taking classes, juggling school, work, and drugs – adding psychedelics to the mix. My attendance suffered and I withdrew.

Needing a new plan, I joined the army. I worked as a surgical technician at Walter Reed Army Medical Center, where I faced daily pressure in the OR.

After four years, I left the Army and continued working in surgery as a member of a trauma/transplant team on night shift at a Portland hospital.

I chose to continue with martial arts and weightlifting.

The night shifts had slower moments, until one night changed everything.

On Father's Day 1987, while working, I was attacked by someone trying to steal narcotics. They struck me from behind with a blunt object, fracturing my skull from the base to around my left ear. I was in a coma for three days, given only a 5% chance of survival.

The next 18 months were filled with overwhelming stress. The brain injury left me unable to do basic math, find the right words, or feel safe. I'd stay up until after 1 a.m. every night – the time of the attack.

My emotional control was gone. I could laugh, cry, or rage without warning. It terrified me and those around me. I went to program for traumatic brain injuries. There, I learned how to rebuild my life. With a team of specialists, I created a program that included memory and concentration exercises, physical activity, positive self-talk, and goal setting.

It was a great addition to my mindfulness practices. I chose to start reading books by Tony Robbins, Wayne Dyer, Deepak Chopra, and Andrew Weil to understand more about the body-mind connection.

I learned that it's more important to respond to situations rather than to react to them. Reacting requires no thought. Response requires a choice.

As part of my recovery, I retrained for a new career in Computer-Assisted Drafting at a local community college. This led to a job at the Bonneville Power Administration.

Eventually, I started questioning my work's purpose. Was I really helping people? I missed the meaning I had found in healthcare.

But a door opened. My brother-in-law offered me a job at his hearing aid business in New Mexico. It sounded like a dream: good pay, a nice house, a fulfilling career. My wife and I decided to go for it.

And then Easter Sunday came.

I had lived through trauma, fear, and years of internal chaos. But through martial arts, meditation, learning, and deep personal work, I found a way to move forward. Stress may never fully leave my life but over the years, I have developed the tools to meet it head-on.

The shift to life in a wheelchair meant that every part of our family dynamics changed. Parenting, shopping, cooking, housekeeping, and even driving had to be adapted. My kids were now my caregivers, my spouse juggled caregiving and being a partner, and my parents and brothers struggled to find where they fit. It was an emotional rollercoaster for all of us.

While reviewing medical records from my court case, I had read physician depositions that revealed the medications I'd been prescribed would likely shorten my life by 10–15 years. I was taking 12–15 pills four times a day, indefinitely. Determined to change course, I worked with my doctor and weaned off all medications within a year – and I actually felt better.

One of the biggest opportunities came when I was invited to join the board of the Oregon Chapter of the Paralyzed Veterans of America (PVA). That led to roles as Hospital Liaison, Vice President, and eventually President. I worked closely with VA hospitals in Seattle and Portland, state and federal legislators, and other national leaders to improve care for veterans and people with disabilities as well as make changes within the VA medical system

After a few years, I resigned to enroll in the Counseling program at Portland State University. As part of my degree, I wrote a 100+ page thesis on the link between diet and depression.

Following my graduation, I ran a successful private practice for ten years focused on people with stress, anxiety, PTSD, and depression.

Based on techniques that I had used all my life, I developed a system using Mindfulness-based stress reduction (MBSR) and Acceptance and Commitment Therapy (ACT) for use with my clients. It's built on the evidence-based practices of Jon Kabat-Zinn, Steven C. Hayes, and Bessel van der Kolk.

It's focused on the neuroscience of stress and anxiety. It teaches you that the thoughts you focus on can change your brain chemistry and how you feel. My clients learned that the anxiety was not their fault; it was their default. The fight-or-flight system was turned on by their thoughts about their situation.

From the success that my clients had with their stress, I authored a book about the 12-stage process titled Living Less Stressed: Keeping Calm in the Chaos.

My personal use of mindfulness and body awareness over the years has helped me through numerous medical issues including four episodes of pressure sores that kept me in bed from 6 to 9 months each time, a case of MRSA (up to 53% death rate), four or five episodes of sepsis (up to 56% death rate), and numerous urinary tract infections.

It has relieved the anxiety of being isolated in bed for months at a time and it has helped me to monitor my physical condition.

Mindfulness helped me choose responses instead of reactions. In a way, it's like taking medication. If you're responding to medication, that's good. If you're reacting to medication, that's bad.

I've learned that words have power. The influence can be positive or negative. It depends on what words you use. The thoughts in your head are words too.

As I look back on my life, did I keep my word in the promise to my father?

I think I did.

After 30+ years of being sentenced to the electric chair, here's a brief list of what I've done to keep that promise.

- Continue the loving relationship with my wife. Our 50th anniversary is next year.

- Raised my sons to be outstanding young men and they run their own businesses.
- Became a grandfather to seven wonderful grandchildren.
- Became a member of Rotary Club, Elks club, and Chamber of Commerce.
- Guest speaker and keynote speaker at several regional events
- Author of numerous national magazine articles
- Recipient of grant from Paralyzed Veterans of America Education Foundation
- Rotarian of the Year, Rotary Club of Oregon City
- President of Rotary Club of Oregon City Foundation
- Member of several honor societies
- Recipient of multiple scholarships
- University Award for Excellence, Portland State University
- Master's Degree in Counselor Education, Portland State University
- Adjunct Instructor, Portland State University
- Shodan Black Belt, American Jujitsu Institute
- Gold medal, Powerlifting, National Veterans Wheelchair Games
- Gold medal, Bowling, National Veterans Wheelchair Games
- President of Oregon chapter of Paralyzed Veterans of America
- Hospital Liaison for Oregon chapter of Paralyzed Veterans of America
- Member of several county advisory councils
- Became a licensed professional counselor and ran a successful private practice for 10 years
- Certified as an Equine-Facilitated Psychotherapist
- Wrote a self-help book titled Living Less Stressed: Keeping Calm in the Chaos, for people with anxiety or PTSD

- Member of The Outlier Project (TOP)
- Became a Life Coach for Stress at Living Less Stressed
- Co-Authored We Choose To Be More Than Our Diagnoses

But I'm not done yet.

My remaining desires include writing a mindfulness cookbook called Stress-cipes; making a mindfulness cartoon strip featuring twin brothers, Les Strest and Max Strest, and setting up an online mindfulness course.

Even though I still can't walk, I can still move forward.

Never let your circumstances dictate what you are capable of doing.

My book 'Living Less Stressed: Keeping Calm in the Chaos' is full of helpful ideas to relieve your stress and anxiety.

Get your copy or sign up for coaching at www.LivingLessStressed.com

BIO:

Jerry Ryan is a Life Coach for Stress and Anxiety, a certified professional with a master's degree in counseling. He is also the author of Living Less Stressed: Keeping Calm in the Chaos, a mindfulness-based guide to finding peace and purpose in uncertain times.

Jerry's life is a testament to resilience. Having survived two major traumatic brain injuries and living for over 30 years as a person with quadriplegia, he understands firsthand what it means to live beyond a diagnosis. His mission is to help people find hope and healing no matter what they're going through, especially those dealing with physical or mental struggles.

Earning a black belt with the American Jujitsu Institute in 2014, Jerry has continued to break barriers throughout his life. He's a longtime advocate for fellow veterans, having served as president of the Oregon chapter of the Paralyzed Veterans of America and as a board member of the Paralyzed Veterans of America Education Foundation. In 2023, at the age of 67, he earned three gold medals at the National Veterans Wheelchair Games, proving that determination and mindset can lead to greatness at any stage of life.

Jerry lives in Oregon City, Oregon, with his wife Marcy, his partner of nearly 50 years. Through his coaching, speaking, and writing, Jerry empowers others to reduce stress, live mindfully, and rise above their limitations. He shows them that calm and courage can coexist in even the most chaotic times.

RE-WIRED
by Joshua MacLeod

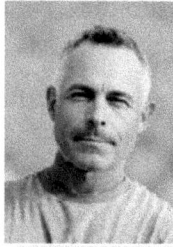

It was supposed to have been a normal day like any other. There were no indications of any danger, no hair standing on end, no gut feeling, no warnings whatsoever. Nothing pointing toward trouble over the horizon. What happened next changed the rest of my life, and little did I know that the hardships, the trials and tribulations I had endured as a child, teen and young adult had prepared me for the biggest challenge of my life. I had never been one to turn away from a challenge, but I was not prepared for the events I am about to relate to you. Carbon monoxide poisoning was a thief that sneaked into my life, and caused me a severe traumatic brain injury. My memory was wiped clean like a white sheet of paper, becoming the ultimate challenge I had to conquer. Most people, when hearing of carbon monoxide poisoning, oftentimes think suicide. Honestly, I can't blame them, as that has become a talking point in modern times. In my case, that was not so, but rather the fault of a negligent third party. Little did I know, I was quite simply an innocent bystander.

The first indication was a severe headache followed by hot spells, and when I glanced in the mirror, my face was flushed red and looked as if I had fallen asleep in the sun. The irony was that no desire of exiting the building arose, as there was no odor or visible indication something was wrong. Hours later, I felt as if my heart was going to explode from within my chest. It was pumping at a rate and force that I never knew possible. Fear-driven, I called my brother and left him a voice message that I was not feeling well and that I was sure I was going to die. I reminded him that he knew what to do and where all the paperwork was stored. I dropped the phone and then went to the corner of the room and dropped to the floor, then everything went quiet and black.

I woke up on a gurney, firefighters rushing me into the back of an ambulance. The medic flashed a light into my eyes as another monitored my heart rate and turned up the oxygen pouring into me through the oxygen mask. They were asking questions, but I could not answer. Everything became black and white. I felt like a lonely buoy swaying in the open ocean with the currents with no land visible. A glimpse of the blue sky flashed across my eyes as they rushed me into the ER. When my eyes opened again, I saw my family as if it were a dream, and then I rolled back into the darkness.

In order for the doctors to get an accurate reading of the amount of carbon monoxide in my blood system, they had to extract a sample from a large artery, not a vein in my arm. Needless to say, I have first-hand experience of being punctured with a large-gauge needle and syringe. When one can see the inside of a needle in its entirety, that is a very large needle. It hurt and hurt bad, but was something I had to endure multiple times within twenty-four hours until the carbon monoxide level in my blood was at 0%. The first sample of blood revealed that I had a carbon monoxide level of 32%. The ER doctor calculated that it was safe to assume that by the time the fire department pulled me out of the building, placed me on pure oxygen and rushed me to the ER, I could have easily been above 40%, if not higher. The doctors at the ER explained that the real side effects would arrive two weeks later, as that was the standard MO across the board.

I felt perfectly fine, and even energized and ready to go, due to being pumped full of fresh oxygen for twenty-four hours straight. They warned me to be careful and not second-guess the effects of carbon monoxide poisoning. The hospital room was quiet, almost too quiet, and when my eyes opened again, I heard two nurses whispering just outside the door, and was surprised when they referred to me as "that's the guy." Apparently, my story had spread throughout the hospital staff as the guy who survived a severe dosage of carbon monoxide poisoning that no one else has. Staff from every level of the hospital were coming in just to look at the face of the man that survived death. I can't tell you how many times I heard, "That's the guy." There was a moment that I felt more like a circus attraction than a patient.

Due to the severe level of carbon monoxide in my blood system, there was technically no cure or treatment because no one had come back from such a severe dose and lived to tell about it. Eventually, I was released from the hospital as a subtle nervousness settled within my head, pondering the approaching two-week deadline. No matter how well I felt, nothing could quell the festering thoughts in the back of my head with each passing day. After week one, I was in denial. I felt great and wanted to put it all behind me and move on.

I met with the attorney who specialized in carbon monoxide poisoning. I remember the look on his face when he read the doctor's report. He dropped into his chair, leaned back and glanced at me with disbelief.

He said he had never met anyone who survived anything over 11%. Noticeable shock showed across his face. He went on to explain that runners and bicyclists along the streets, around cars or within city limits ingest an average of 3% to 5% carbon monoxide and never even know it. Chain smokers have an average of 6% to 8% in their blood daily. People die of carbon monoxide poisoning between 9% and 11%, depending on their health. Anything above 12% is fatal. He suggested I start with hyperbaric chamber treatments, ASAP. Needless to say, he took the case.

Into week two, I felt normal and was starting to put aside any thoughts or fears and also declined starting hyperbaric chamber treatments, but it all changed one day shy of the full two-week deadline when I woke up to a blank mind that felt empty and hollow. I had no memory of who I was or where I was. I had a distinct awkward feeling that I was an organism in a petri dish with no purpose. I was alive, but where and how? There was an awareness that I could breathe and I could feel. At the time, those were such bizarre feelings, as my mind was totally devoid of any memories.

The room was bright-white as fresh snow, and it seemed as if it went on forever in every direction. I was lying in a bed with no memory. None at all. I remember standing and glancing around, trying to find an answer to my existence, but nothing came to mind. Only bright-white haunted me in every direction I glanced. Thankfully, memories occasionally would come flooding back in bits and pieces. It was those unexpected glimpses of hope, of normalcy, that I would take advantage of, and started implementing my rehab and comeback with sticky notes and photos, which became my daily friends in a world of sudden uncertainty. It was the slow, painful start of a long and painful rehabilitation. I had suddenly found myself on a deserted island, and I was the single occupant.

Thankfully, I leaned upon the experience I had being a gym rat and working out. I had competed in marathons and was an avid jogger and always ate healthy and stayed fit. My lifestyle was hardcore workouts, and they were normal for me, as pain is weakness leaving the body. I had some friends that were professional bodybuilders, so I had a level of understanding of what type of dedication and discipline I had to focus on to succeed and overcome the handicap that I was facing.

When I had moments of clarity, the fear of being handicapped would drive me forward to fight. My notes reminded me who I was and what I needed to do, and explained what I did the previous day. They were reminders to work out, to eat, to shower, to brush my teeth, to read and so forth and so forth. My notes reminded me to play catch with a tennis ball against the wall to help with reflexes, as my depth perception was so poor that I couldn't even catch the ball. I dropped coffee mugs and plates simply because my mind couldn't gauge distances, and everything felt like an optical illusion, causing me to second-guess every move I made. Thus, a large number of plates, mugs and cups ended in pieces on the floor. My head, shoulders, arms and legs were covered in bruises due to walking into walls, doors and doorframes, even though my mind and eyes said I was clear. My speech became slurred and I stuttered with great annoyance. Time became opaque because it slipped by so fast, only because I would fade away into a white world with no depth. This is only a short version of a long story, but it is a reminder of how far I had come. When my doctors suggested they could write me a prescription for a handicapped decal and rearview mirror plaque, I refused. The thought of being labeled as handicapped was so intense that I could not even imagine it. "No" was my final answer.

The daily routine was the same: start over from scratch and keep going. Each passing day recycled itself into the next as the routines were replicated. Eventually, I graduated from playing tennis ball against wall and picked up playing video games to improve my cognitive response time. Video games were never my thing, in fact, I frowned upon them because I felt they were making our kids dumb and violent. It was a two-edged sword that I had to juggle, and to my surprise, things improved for me on many levels as the fast pace of the video games forced my mind to think, and most of all, react. Personally, without any scientific evidence, I can say with certainty that I started seeing a dramatic change, as the video games were an unexpected game-changer; no pun intended. I had a unique feeling that my brain was healing itself in a way that I could not understand at the time, but I knew something was happening. I had the odd feeling that the fastest way to succeed was to start and figure it out along the way because I couldn't learn to drive a parked car.

Thanks to my mother, I started daily hyperbaric chamber treatments for six months straight. My mother maxed out her credit card just to get me help, as she believed the hyperbaric chamber would bring, and she was right; it did! To this day, I attribute most of my success to the hyperbaric chamber. The hour-long sessions I spent in those chambers forced 100% oxygen into my blood and thus helped my brain re-wire itself. I cannot explain how my mind re-wired itself, but I can say that I'm a totally different man than before. Still on the hunt for a cure, I took every day as a chance to continue searching and trying.

A threshold appeared after a few months, and it was clear to me that I had a long way to go before I could move to the next level. I hit a wall of depression and felt as if I were dead. There were always two people in the room fighting for the same space. Those feelings were formidable, and I couldn't shake them off. Thoughts of hopelessness, anxiety and not having a purpose raced through my head like a squirrel in a wheel. Navigating through the constant bombardment had become a daily fight to say the least. It was a dark place for me, as I was suffering both mentally and physically, as if a noose had been placed around my neck and I was gasping for air. Therein was the problem. The old me had died and I couldn't do anything about it. It took me a long time to accept the fact that I had to let go of the old me, cut the line and let him sink into the depths of 'what was' and allow the new me to grow and step inside this body and into 'what would become.' There were times I would glance at my arms and down at my body and felt like a ghost in a shell. The disconnect was nightmarish.

Moments of clarity were often enough to help with staying on track with routines and setting goals. It was during one of those moments of clarity when I recalled one of my favorite quotes by Marcus Aurelius: "What stands in the way, becomes the way." And just like that, I realized that I had to embrace my new reality and work with it rather than trying to fix it. I was hellbent on trying to discover a cure that would never come rather than embracing my circumstance. In the mirror, I had a long, difficult and honest conversation with myself. It was brutal and heart-wrenching. I cried and cried until my eyes looked back at me in the mirror when a determined acceptance had settled in, and I knew in my heart that I had torn down a mental wall within myself. I came out of the room a changed man. I had let it all go, like an anchor cut off the deck of a ship now sinking into the darkness beneath.

With a new lease on life, I was determined to overcome this handicap rather than hoping I could find a cure. I reached out to my doctors and asked for a prescription for HGH, otherwise known as human growth hormone, because I wanted to take it in conjunction with hyperbaric treatments. As we age, our bodies stop producing HGH, and eventually, that is where our aging sets in. Human growth hormone helps the body heal itself. To my utter disbelief, no doctor wanted to write me a prescription for the HGH, as they said it wouldn't help. They frowned upon anything controversial and homeopathic. In reality, I knew they were scared that it would work but wouldn't verbalize it because their god was science.

Frustrated, I reached out to my friends in the bodybuilding world, and again, thanks to my mom, I bought a six-month supply of HGH. I started taking it once every day and continued with hyperbaric treatments. Within two weeks, I started seeing results. Not only was I sleeping better, I was starting to feel normal and noticing my mind was working again. I was having fewer blank moments and more clarity and was retaining what I was doing and why. It was the first time in months that I was actually seeing I was making substantial progress. There came a realization when I noticed that most people with severe brain injuries were bedridden and didn't move a lot or not at all. I knew that movement was key to circulating the blood, and circulating the blood with a high oxygen content was key to a recovery because I knew the brain needs oxygen to survive. Thus, I concluded that if I could feed my brain a steady dose of fresh oxygen with the HGH, my brain could heal.

My hypothesis was correct. After six months, I was functioning at a level no one expected. So I continued with this routine while increasing my workouts and walking three to five miles per day, as I was using the exercise to increase oxygen intake when not in the hyperbaric chamber. Yes, the video games continued as well as online cognitive exams, and I picked up reading again to help keep my brain on its toes. I wanted to keep my brain busy! Reading was not easy because I was not retaining what I was reading. I had to re-read everything two, three, four or more times to understand what it was I was reading. It was truly a frustrating time. Nonetheless, my brain adapted to the reading and I started enjoying it again. Although I was working out physically, one could argue that I actually had my brain on a steady workout routine, not my body.

It was during this time that I realized I had become left-handed when I was and have always been right-handed. That was when I realized my brain had somehow re-wired itself. I could sign my name with my left hand and could use my left hand as if it were always normal for me. I knew that my dedication had paid off. The belief of feeding my brain as much oxygen as possible was the key to overcoming a severe handicap. Pure oxygenated blood was what helped my brain heal and re-wire itself. I believe this with such an intensity that no one can tell me otherwise. This was my life for the next thirteen years, and I can say that I will continue with what works for me. The only difference is the intensity level is not as intense, but rather now a slow boil of healing.

My journey took me down a long and winding path of self-discovery, discipline and dedication, one I would not change for anything in this world only because I discovered a layer of the human body so few people ever get a glimpse of. It did not come easy, but I'm happy it did arrive, as my journey was only one of many around the world. My advice to those searching for an answer is simple: we have a wealth of information available to us nowadays. Keep searching for your healing and stay busy with what works for you. It's so easy to fall down the trap of victimhood in a day and age that sells victimhood-ism. Don't buy it!

BIO:

Joshua MacLeod is a survivor of severe carbon monoxide poisoning. His recovery was a miracle and one he enjoys sharing with the world. He is the author of 4 books: Savage Tango, Savage House, Savage Seas and Chasing Latitudes, and an eight-year veteran columnist for East Coast Current. He lives on the east coast of Florida with his four dogs, Durango, Higgins, Oscar and Brody.

www.joshuamacleod.com

PAIN, PROGRESS, VICTORY
Surviving the Unthinkable and Finding Purpose in the Pain
by Dr. LaQuita Parks

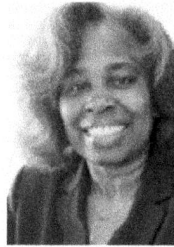

Pain has been a part of my life since I was four years old. And it all started with a simple procedure. Having my tonsils removed started a medical tsunami for me that has lasted for the last 51 years and quite honestly, will last for the rest of my life.

But, I am more than my diagnoses.

I was only four years old when I went into Grady Memorial Hospital in Atlanta, Georgia, to have my tonsils removed. Just a simple procedure, they said, nothing to worry about they said. Kids got their tonsils taken out all the time back then. A little discomfort, some ice cream, and a few days of rest. That's all it was supposed to be. But for me, it became the beginning of a storm that I will spend the rest of my life learning to survive.

The tonsillectomy was a success. That's what they told my mama. That's what the doctors said. That's what everyone believed. I was just four years old, and I had made it through my very first surgery like a little champ. I was supposed to go home the next morning but sometime during the night, a nurse entered my room without much of a word. She carried a tray with a syringe and said she needed to give me a shot. I don't know if any questions were asked or not, all I know is she pulled back my covers and jabbed the needle deep into my right thigh. She struck the nerve!

I screamed and kept screaming. The pain was tremendous.

My right leg began to swell and almost instantly, my leg blew up like a balloon, growing by the second. There was mass chaos. Doctors were suddenly everywhere.

The swelling wouldn't stop. I was rushed into emergency surgery. The doctors told my mother, who walked into the hospital as they were rushing me into surgery that if they didn't act immediately, my leg would burst from the pressure. And if that happened, I could die. They were preparing to amputate my leg.

In the operating room, they opened my leg to release the pressure. What they found was worse than expected. During the eight-hour surgery, they found that instead of removing the entire leg, they could remove the bone. They believed that would save my life—and it did—but it came at a cost. When the surgery was over, they told my mama I would never walk again.

Interestingly enough, the only thing I can remember from that horrible incident is my Uncle Donald coming to see me in the hospital on Christmas. He was dressed like Santa Claus and he carried a bag full of green colored toys. I often wonder why the green toys are the only memory I really have of that time, especially since it has affected my life in such a major way.

Over the years, the theory is I suppressed the memory because it was too traumatic. It still amazes me how the mind has a way of protecting us from things we can't handle. That was the beginning of a new reality.

Fifteen surgeries later on my right leg and foot, I'm still walking. But I've never known a day without pain.

I mean that literally: not one day. Not one morning waking up pain-free. Not one moment completely at ease in my own body. Not one memory of running without limping or standing without balance.

Pain 24 hours a day, 7 days a week for 50 years…600 months, 438, 288 (four hundred thirty-eight thousand, two hundred eighty-eight) hours, 26, 297, 280 (twenty-six million, two hundred ninety-seven thousand, two hundred eighty) minutes and 1, 577, 836, 800 (One billion, five hundred seventy-seven million, eight hundred thirty-six thousand, eight hundred) seconds. Now let me let that sink in for a moment!

That single moment, one careless injection in the middle of the night, rewrote my entire life.

The nurse never came back.

No one ever apologized.

The hospital never took responsibility.

Something had gone terribly wrong—and they buried it under silence and denial.

And while they buried the truth, I was learning how to live with what they left behind:

- Metal braces on my leg.

- Crutches and walkers and physical therapy.

- Shame in school.

- Stares from strangers.

- A childhood shaped by surgeries and scar tissue.

And the pain—always the pain. Physical, emotional, spiritual.

But let me tell you what they didn't bury: me.

I was supposed to lose my leg.

They said I'd never walk.

They said I'd always be limited.

But I kept walking.

Kept moving.

Kept speaking.

Kept believing.

In 2020, I walked into the Mayo Clinic in Jacksonville, Florida, desperate for answers. After decades of pain, procedures, and pushing through life with a body that never quite cooperated, I needed someone to see me. Not just my symptoms. Not just my scars. Me.

The doctors ran every test they could. Bloodwork. Imaging. Physical evaluations. They poked, prodded, and analyzed. I had been through this before, but something about this visit felt different. I didn't want another pill. I didn't want another shrug. I wanted someone to name what had been tormenting me all my life.

When the doctor came into the room, he sat down, looked me in the eyes, and said, "Although you're not dying, you are suffering."

That sentence held both relief and heartbreak.

I wasn't dying—but I wasn't fully living either.

I was surviving pain that never stopped.

Existing in a body that felt like it was constantly under attack.

They gave it names this time:

Lupus. Fibromyalgia. Lymphedema. PTSD. Chronic Pain Syndrome.

I finally had the labels.

But the truth is, those diagnoses didn't define me—they confirmed what I already knew: I was living a life that hurt more than it helped, and yet I kept going anyway.

I am not just a list of conditions.

I am not just what's in my chart or written in bold on the top of a medical report. I am not a case study or a cautionary tale.

I am a woman. A mother. A fighter. A believer.

I am laughter in the middle of a flare-up.

I am tears held back so someone else can feel strong.

I am faith wrapped in flesh that won't always cooperate.

I live with pain—but pain doesn't live in me.

I carry trauma—but trauma doesn't carry me.

I have limitations—but they don't get the last word.

The Mayo Clinic gave me clarity. But what they didn't give me—what no doctor could give me—was the will to live beyond those diagnoses. That part came from somewhere deeper. From God. From grit. From everything I've overcome since the moment that nurse jabbed me in the thigh when I was just a child.

I've learned that suffering can shape you—but it doesn't get to define you.And I'm still here. Still standing.

Not cured. Not whole. Not painless.

But powerful.

Because I am more than my pain.

More than my past.

More than any diagnosis on any piece of paper.

I am purpose.

I am perseverance.

I am proof.

That moment at the Mayo Clinic in 2020—when the doctor looked me in the eyes and acknowledged my suffering—did something to me. It was the first time in a long time that I felt seen beyond the surface. Not just as a patient, but as a woman who had carried more pain than most people could imagine, and still showed up every day trying to make something of it.

The diagnosis didn't free me.

But it did wake me.

I realized then that healing doesn't always come in the form of medicine or surgery. Sometimes, healing comes when you give your pain a voice. When you stop hiding. When you stop pretending you're fine just because everyone else is uncomfortable with the truth.

And that's when the vision for Pa-Pro-Vi Publishing was born.

Pain. Progress. Victory.

That's what the name stands for.

That's what my life has stood for.

Because without pain, I wouldn't have grown.

Without progress, I wouldn't have found my path.

And without both, I would never have found the victory in helping others do the same.

I didn't set out to become a publisher.

I didn't go looking to build a platform.

I was just trying to survive.

But in that space between suffering and surrender, God whispered a new assignment:

"Tell your story. And help others tell theirs."

So I did.

I told the story of that nurse at Grady Hospitalwho almost cost me my leg—and my life. I told the story of surgeries and setbacks, of single motherhood, and of pushing through pain that never asked permission to stay.

And I began helping others share their own journeys—from trauma to testimony.

Every book I publish is more than a project. It's a lifeline.

Every author I work with isn't just a client—they're a survivor too.

Because stories heal. Stories free. Stories restore.

And for many of us, writing is how we breathe when life tries to choke the hope out of us.

Pa-Pro-Vi Publishing isn't just a business. It's a ministry.

A movement.

A legacy.

It started in a hospital room.

It started in silence and pain.

But it lives on in pages, in people, in purpose.

And if you're holding this book, reading these words, and feeling like maybe your pain has a purpose too—believe me when I say:

It does.

Your story matters.

Your voice matters.

You matter.

There are days when I wake up and the pain is so loud, I can barely hear my own thoughts.

Before my feet even hit the floor, it's there—aching, pulsing, wrapping itself around my body like an old enemy that refuses to leave. Some mornings, I lie still with tears on my pillow, whispering prayers not for healing, but for strength just to endure one more day.

Because this pain doesn't take a break.

It doesn't clock out.

It doesn't ask permission to show up in the middle of a task, a dream, a moment of joy. It just is—relentless.

But so is my faith.

If you ask me how I've made it this far—how I've endured over fifty years of physical pain, emotional trauma, and spiritual warfare—the answer is simple:

God.

It's not a cliché for me.

It's not something I say just to sound strong.

It's the truth.

Every step I take—every single one—is an act of faith.

Every smile I give is a prayer in motion.

Every book I help someone publish, every coaching session, every hug, every word I write—it's all covered in grace. Because I know I don't move on my own. I never have.

Pain may have taken pieces of my body, but it could never steal my spirit.

That belongs to God.

There were nights I cried myself to sleep asking "Why me?"

And mornings I woke up angry that I was still here, still hurting, still fighting to put on my clothes, comb my hair, and show up in the world like I wasn't breaking inside.

But even in those moments—especially in those moments—God never left me.

His presence met me in the hospital room when the nurse disappeared. He was with me through every surgery, every scar, every unanswered question. He held me when doctors spoke limitations over my life.

And He reminded me: "I'm not finished with you yet."

See, faith doesn't always take the pain away.

But it gives the pain purpose.

I've learned to look at my pain differently.

Not as a punishment, but as a platform. A platform to encourage. To uplift. To help someone else see that they're not alone in their suffering.

My faith is not passive—it's active.

It walks with me. It breathes through me.

It holds me up when my legs want to give out—physically and spiritually.

The Bible says in 2 Corinthians 12:9,

"My grace is sufficient for you, for my power is made perfect in weakness."

That verse isn't just scripture to me. It's my life.

Because when I am weak—and believe me, I have known weakness—His strength shows up stronger than anything I could ever muster on my own.

Yes, I have Lupus.

Yes, I have Fibromyalgia, Lymphedema, PTSD, and chronic pain.

Yes, I have scars.

But I also have faith.

And my faith reminds me daily:

I may be walking with a limp, but I am still walking.

I may cry, but I am still called.

I may ache, but I still have anointing.

I am not forgotten. I am favored.

I don't know what tomorrow holds.

But I know Who holds me.

And as long as I have breath in my body, I will keep showing up—limping, pressing, praying, and praising.

Because **my story is not about pain.**

It's about victory through faith.

For many years I have struggled with one type of pain or another. I have had to deal with physical pain along with emotional pain holding its hand. Pain is a serious thing. It can make you or break you. It can stop you dead in your tracks or push you forward, full speed ahead. Pain can totally derail you or totally define you. Instead of letting my pain derail or define me, I chose to trust God and allow Him to re-define me.

A good friend of mine once told me that I have the tenacity of a pit bull on steroids. After I finished laughing, I had to know why he described me this way. He responded that I had an amazing capacity to endure whatever came my way. As I think about it, I guess you can say my capacity to endure like a pit bull on steroids began the day I was born.

To say that I had the power to choose my course in life was a foreign concept to me then because I was just a little girl, and no one taught me that there could be more to my life than what I was enduring. Although I was young, I was very weak and from my perspective, there were no aspects of my life that I was looking forward to. The game for me then was survival. The game for me now is vitality, growth, and development.

Life was tough for me but there was something inside of me that would not allow me to quit, no matter how difficult things got. As I got older, I started to realize that there was healing in sharing, so I started to share my story. I also began to recognize that I was behaving like a victim (even though I was), I had the power to be victorious, but only if I chose to be. I didn't like people to pity me because it made me feel like I was a weak link, so I became even more determined.

There was nothing I could do about my condition, what happened to me was not my fault and I could have sat down and had myself quite the pity party, but I wanted more for my life. I wanted a quality life. I knew that the power to live and thrive was a choice and I wanted to make it.

I want the world to know that you can do anything you want to do. You become what you focus on the most. If you say you can't, then you won't. But if you say you can, then you certainly will. I am fifty-five years old and have lived with chronic pain since I was four years old. Every day I make the choice to live and if that means I have the tenacity of a pit bull on steroids, then I will take it because… I am more than my diagnoses!

BIO:

Dr. LaQuita Parks (Hon.) is the Founder and CEO of **Pa-Pro-Vi Publishing** and **A Failure 2 Communicate LLC**, as well as an **8x International Best-Selling Author, Relationship Communication Coach, Writing Coach, Motivational Speaker, and Mentor** with an unwavering passion for people and their well-being.

Dr. LaQuita received her **Doctor of Humane Letters (Honoris Causa)** and the **Credential of Global Fellowship in Leadership Principles** from Mainseed Christian University. She is also a **2024 Presidential Lifetime Achievement Award** recipient, a **2024 It's In A Book Award** honoree, and was named **2022 Making Headline News Woman of the Year**. Additionally, she received the **Trivia's Inspirational Radio Community Excellence Award, and Making Headline News Woman of the Year Award** in 2022. As the host of two impactful podcast shows, **"My Heart on Pages"** and **"So, What's Your Story"**, LaQuita provides a platform for meaningful storytelling and healing. She has been a **contributing writer and sponsor** for I Am International Magazine since 2021 and is also a **contributing writer** for the award-winning Listen Linda magazine.

Since launching **Pa-Pro-Vi Publishing** in 2020, LaQuita has **coached hundreds of authors worldwide**, guiding them from **"thought to realization"** in their storytelling journey. She has successfully **published over 150 solo book projects for various authors**, with more than half achieving **Amazon Bestseller** status, and nearly **20 anthologies**, most of which have become bestsellers. In total, she has collaborated with over **400 contributing authors**. Additionally, LaQuita has authored multiple books, including two **co-authored children's books**.

Contact Dr. LaQuita at www.paprovipublishing.com

RENDING CHOICES
by Lydia Lowery Busler

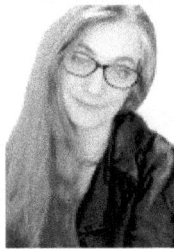

Everyone has darkness in them. Whatever light we hold, the darkness promises power, the drama of stealth, and the whisper of security. And while some gravitate toward the light, some wax unabashedly darkward. Still others simply hold such unwavering fascination with either dark or light that they see no choice.

Darkness holds a key. No one can touch us or hold us to any norms there. What if the darkness is only stunning because we're so bright? We may be on the precipice of a breakthrough we'll never see because we've built a fortress where we are.

When darkness becomes overwhelming, there's a rend in our belief, in our very being. We feel more than pain. We feel we're being torn asunder.

I've felt agony like that, when regardless of what I'd previously believed, I did an about-face in light of pain's incredulity. I could have reacted with anger and stayed stuck. But I learned that, in my continued defiance, my life took a very different course than had I surrendered to a diagnosed expectation.

Defiance insists we witness the feeling. When pain passes a threshold that shifts reality, defiance becomes a sort of self-love, present in the feeling. Accepting the pain in our presence.

Refusal to accept the story behind the pain is where the wild transformative wonders are. Curiosity about unseen truth opens up a lot of possibilities. When we release blame and spite, instead embracing self-responsive defiance of the prevaling story, we thrust ourselves so forcefully into a different light that we defy our malady altogether.

Utter defiance has torn me open and shone a light on my inner power, forgiveness, and the transformative qualities of surrender. Life without challenge is stagnant, and stagnation isn't synonymous with life.

I don't consider the chapters of pain in my life in chronological order. They're more like a freight train. If I attach myself to the noise, it's overwhelming. If I get on the train and ride, it's quieter and I can participate and see it through.

Everything is a story. Everything.

So many stories sweep us away in a strong current of cultural momentum. They imprint us with mental scotomas - literal blind spots which obliterate our ability to comprehend anything not already in our belief system. We can't see anything, and before we know it, we've discredited our own dreams.

But dreams change, we can change, and our beliefs change when we become curious and aware of the universal truth in all we've experienced and learned. It's in that curiosity where the story becomes poised to shift. I've had counselors, therapists, psychologists, and psychiatrists my whole life, and there was a tale for each. Some listened deeply and curiously to my stories, drawing tales out like a passionate professor of fiction. Some asked pointed questions, probing that which didn't seem congruent with their concept of a complete human being. Some, early on, were on a set path for truth, honesty, and justice, and if something didn't make sense to their truth, it was deemed dishonest. I learned there and then how to craft a story that released me from their services quickly and assured a future of more self-exploration.

Diagnoses stacked - CPTSD, ADHD, TBI, Chronic Atypical Migraine, Asplenia, Depression, and neurodivergencies I delighted in discovering later. They've been a steady part of my life, misunderstood by those who've not been tortured, maimed, altered by brain injuries, or been in hospitals so long that every patient on the floor either went home or died. Diagnoses become a way of life, shading how we negotiate each new challenge, microaggressions stacking in accordance with our adaptive trauma response.

Moving in life toward a space where the air is more breathable is a practice in which vision continuously becomes clearer and brighter, more and more splendid. I'm never done. And that's beautiful.

In my memory, there was no story in the beginning, only my curiosity and questioning what and why and how. My story began there, and my world was full of woods and music. I sang before I talked. Music has always been my first language. In the woods, I connected to the trees, plants, and wildlife. Telepathy was my second language, and this is my first story.

My sweet, creative nature seemed to attract an attention that was under oath of silence. Abuse by so many people became a way of life, robbing me daily of sleep, removing my gentle boundaries. I was waterboarded and virginity taken over and over. I found solace in art, in the woods, and in the agony
and ecstasy of music.

I can't even recall when it started; it was just the unfolding of life, perplexing and overwhelming interactions interspersed with the unwavering support of trees.

Music and trees are connected. Music is made of distinct pitches. They're not the same if produced with another vibration, even if they're relative to one another. I seemed to possess an unusual 'absolute pitch' which simply made sense to me. Just as leaves on one plant aren't the same leaves as on another, a red dress by a designer isn't the same as a blue dress by that designer. Further, musical pitches correspond to the earth, flavored with moss and minerals and colored as distinctly as crayons in a crayon box. I never understood people who couldn't grasp what I was saying. If they could name different colors, why couldn't they name pitches?

Music became something easy and intrinsic for me. I played the horn and spent a great deal of time with it. All the language I needed was there, and it was all positive and spoke deeply to my soul.

And then there was school. Academia was a place of both ease and discomfort. Expectation of perfect grades, no rest, and not-yet-diagnosed neurodivergence brought a thick sense of separation without understanding why.

After about ten years, I reported my abuse. I found an enormous well of compassion for my abusers whom I gleaned had been abused themselves. They showed love and tried to make me strong in the messed-up ways they knew how. I forgave them. Deeply. In forgiveness, I waded into a pool of healing for myself.

A bazaar car crash started a new chapter in my life. Driving to work on a back road after a thaw in March, my water jug wobbled on the passenger seat as I rounded a corner. My next brief memory is of the rearview mirror shattered and my face obliterated by blood. I had no idea who I was, but I said to that cracked mirror,

"Wow, you look horrible." I would know myself by my inner judgment.

By some stroke of grace, there was an EMT on the road 10 minutes behind me. My car was found accordioned, the speedometer frozen at 40 mph, between a big oak tree with an oil stain 4 feet up its trunk, and a mailbox that was eerily untouched. There was a single ridge of ice on the road behind. All anyone can figure is that I hit that ridge of ice and was airborne and flew over that mailbox and into that tree.

I was rushed from one hospital to the next and then died oh-so-quietly on the operating table shortly after being intubated while awake. Honestly, death is lovely. Death is not suffering, it's peace. I felt held, not accosted, with no concept of worry.

But evidently, it wasn't my time, and in retrospect, that was a strange disappointment. I held the serene memory of death like a blissful, abundant sleep, returned to human consciousness, and acquiesced to a pain that presented like an open window on survival and humanity itself.

My spleen and pancreas had been pulverized. Insulin and amylase are made in the pancreas. It's incredibly vital, and when compromised, leaks an abundance of caustic, acidic proteins. Healthy amylase levels are around 30-60 U/L. My blood amylase was above 3000 U/L, so an onslaught of desperate acts to halt its production ensued to stop it from digesting my whole body from within.

I'm grateful for my time in the hospital. I learned the meaning of true care and a lot about both ego, service, helplessness, and rescue. I had plenty of time, sleepless nights, and stories in that hospital as I stabilized through several surgeries. I couldn't eat, drink, or even have liquid touch my lips for three months. But when I walked out, I could begin to taste food anew. I also had stretchy, new skin on a repaired face, a traumatic brain injury, a weird feeling where my spleen used to be, a tender third of my pancreas, an altered colon, and an oddly floppy knee that mostly righted itself laying around for months. I slowly reentered society with my compromised immune system, brain, and digestion, and a keen sense of 4am.

It took a while for me to work out my incessant awkwardness in the world, and this new altered anatomy was too much to hope to explain to anyone. I gently but swiftly worked myself back into shape.

The music industry turned out to be misogynistic as ever upon my reentry, no better to reinstate tender boundaries I desperately needed. I took to the sidewalks and beat them with my fists, mourning all those suffering in dark places, a loud - shamefully loud - behavior. And I buried myself in my music.

It wasn't until a college jury audition, just months after leaving the hospital, that my internal perception of my true self was challenged. I was asked to perform a prepared work, which was acclaimed by the jury, but when I was asked to sight read a new piece of music, I couldn't do it, and I was shamed for it.

Simply mortified, I promised myself never to allow that to happen again in my life. I set out training myself to sight read very well. Honestly, having performed Principal Horn with Yo Yo Ma and the Boston Symphony Orchestra when I was sixteen for the grand opening of the Hynes Convention Center created very high expectations for myself. I worked my way through a number of colleges to make things right.

One day, all that came to an awkward halt as I walked down the street and my knee crumpled. Turned out that the Posterior Cruciate ligament (PCL) in my knee had been hanging on by a thread since my car crash, but since I'd brought myself back very slowly and built up my thigh muscles biking, hiking, and cross-country skiing, I never realized anything was wrong. It felt stable until the thread snapped.

The surgeon I chose had completed his doctoral thesis specifically on PCL surgery, though he'd never actually performed the surgery; it had only ever been completed about 20 times out on the West Coast of the United States (I was on the East Coast at the time). The surgeon offered to refer me to a doctor out west, but as I explored options, it turned out the procedure had been redone on each western patient, so I opted to trust him and stay. Simultaneous for surgery, I had the good fortune to place in the finals for a huge international performance competition. I looked forward to donning a new knee for this upcoming music test in Europe.

On the morning of surgery, prone on the table, anesthetic was administered into my IV while I faced someone who was not the same anesthesiologist I had met pre-op. I had an eerie, alarmed feeling about this guy, judging him harshly at the gut level before I nodded off into a very long slumber.

I woke from eleven hours of surgery, terribly nauseated, with my mom nearby and a nurse saying, "I've never seen a tourniquet left on that long." I shrugged it off, too close to being sick over the side of the bed to care.

My leg was the size of a midwest city and I shrugged that off, too, since this was all new territory. The leg stayed swollen for two weeks. At the end of those two weeks, a long nightmare took hold.

The leg was gone, atrophied down to a wisp of bone. Where my beautiful leg muscles once lived was a seering, wet, fiendish pain. That first day was utterly perplexing, like I was being stabbed through the bottom of my foot up to my knee with a wet, slightly warm blade exactly 3/16" thick and 1.5" wide, over and over. I couldn't eat and I couldn't sleep for the next two weeks, all I could do was scream.

The anesthesiologist feigned a weak attempt to diagnose me, administering a random lumbar block and prescribing enormous amounts of percocet. No one knew what had happened except for that nurse from post-op. Expecting something was amiss, she obtained my records for me and explained how they work:

An anesthesiologist is responsible for the tourniquet. The tourniquet keeps the blood out of the surgeon's way, and loosening it at regular intervals allows enough blood to keep the limb alive. The records indicated that the tourniquet had been removed periodically for the first four hours, but after that, remained tight for the remaining seven hours.

Meanwhile, the surgeon had been doing the cutting and restringing, concentrating only on his job.

I ended up sending my records to a big malpractice law firm, communicating with them daily. They seemed keen to focus on the terrible negligence and huge blow to my career path.

Then one day, they didn't call. Another day passed. And another. When I reached out for a progress report, they seemed to have completely forgotten me. They gradually feigned vague remembrance.

"Oh, that bum leg, yes, you don't have a case," they asserted offhandedly.

Huh? What about my records?
"Your records show nothing abnormal."

I requested my original records back. When they arrived - the records were altered. Furious, I inquired at the hospital for the nurse who had cared for me and helped obtain the records.

She was nowhere to be found. There was no record of her ever having worked at the hospital. She no longer existed.

A neurologist next certified that all of my motor, sympathetic, and sensory nerves and their sheaths were dead from the hip socket down. While I could maybe grow back a small bit of nerves because I was still in my 20s, they only grow ⅛" a year at best and the neurologist posited I'd be lucky to regain half an inch. He maintained that it was unlikely the pain would stop and there was nothing for me to do but pain management.

There was an uproar. Everyone in my inner circle was incensed. My family insisted I sue the lawyer as well as the anesthesiologist. My husband suggested assisted suicide. Then something shifted hard in me. My spirit took over and there was no ego in the way anymore. I saw myself in the garden, bare feet, whole and mobile. My spirit spoke.

"No. There's nothing wrong with me. I can walk."

That moment changed my life. I spent the next year-and-a-half screaming as I made myself walk with daily physical therapy, acupuncture, and a whole lot of raw eggs. I grew three feet of nerves, around a meter, in 18 months.

What I didn't know then is that the brain can't accept cognitive dissonance, and I wouldn't accept defeat. My declaration set into motion a sweeping manifestation, and my mind helped everything fall into place. It's simple - I chose to heal. It was medically impossible. (If people could grow nerves that fast with raw eggs, they'd all be doing it.) But I did it.

I'll never be defined by the stories of the trauma in my life. Every rending choice I've made had no guarantees but the certainty of my own belief. My belief. I won't let that be defined by anyone else.

I missed out on that competition. But once I completed getting degreed, I played Principal Horn once again, this time in the Opera di Roma in Italy before moving to New York City and playing in the NYC Ballet and for the Jose Limon Dancers. I was even invited and groomed for the highest paying horn job in the world at the time by the Metropolitan Opera Orchestra.

I loved the Met. That's another story, one of the suspension of doubt and embrace of the fantastic and otherworldly. But I was pregnant with my son and I opted out of the audition. I always assumed it was the pregnancy and the ex-husband that caused me to walk away. While that was partially true, it also may have been a good thing. It distanced me from a great deal of the male-dominated, inappropriate world of orchestral music, and I went on to become a solo improvisationalist on my own terms.

It's funny how we just keep learning. Years later, a non-musician friend talked about her experience with something called synesthesia, and that's when I realized that I'm also a synesthete. It seems that synesthesia, a cross-perception of senses, isn't part of the cultural narrative. The discovery led me to understand something that had troubled me before: while early in life, I could read music and had a fantastic ear, I always heard the music with all its associated tastes and colors before I read it. Looking back, when I was asked to sight read in front of that jury long before, there were no colors. There were no minerals. There were only black notes. I was utterly blind when I failed. What I unwittingly had done after that which was so unusual was to teach myself to read the black notes and understand how they sounded, appeared, and tasted from what I read.

Back then, I had also taken some time in the culinary arts as a chef (and later worked in wine), and that was a fantastic place for my unrealized synesthesia to shine when working with people I served. But I didn't stay there, I started a private music studio and can see now that all of my descriptive, intuitive, synesthetic ways also worked very well for teaching.

Stories wended and wove as I got my pace in life.

I gave birth. It was different because of adhesions that were a part of my core, but I didn't know the difference. I experienced deep awe, filtered through synesthesia and understanding of death, but I didn't know the difference.

I traveled as an orchestral and improvisational performer, and the music I wrote reached the far corners of the world. It still does. I'm grateful.

I lost track of my limbs, my vision flipped backward, and my brain forgot how to speak and left me wordless, a symptom laced with an anguish I long judged in myself. Now, I have the help of a neurological team and baseline shots for life.

I get yearly immunizations to stave off diseases no one else gets. I don't digest without pharmaceutical enzymes at every meal. I understand all this because my body was chipped away and blown apart and parts were reinstalled, wabi-sabi kintsugi. Shots and therapy are the love and the glue.

I forgive again and again. In forgiveness, my life is in my own hands, without energy in blame. I follow the path of love and awe. Connecting to the air, the trees, the sea, and grounding in nature brings the requisite stillness to be present with pain and transformation, a calm which now sustains me.

Every darkness is the catalyst for a new brightness.

BIO:
From overcoming life-threatening injuries and defying medical odds to gracing stages with the Boston Symphony, Opera di Roma, Jose Limon Dancers, and New York City Ballet, my path constantly reveals our

extraordinary potential as humans to heal ourselves. As a composer, performer, and improvisational artist with records and productions all over the world, I've spent my life creating transformative experiences through music and earning induction into the ACME International Hall of Fame.

What has emerged is that I love empowering others to heal and thrive. After rebuilding my own body and spirit time after time, I became fascinated by the unseen healing journey. I followed my curiosity and studied with pioneers in mental fitness, healing, and coaching, integrating diverse methods into a comprehensive and dynamic healing approach. As founder of The Joyful Path LLC, I guide individuals and groups toward mind-body-soul alignment to foster clarity, heal, and attain "Jedi calm."

So now, I help stressed professionals and creatives unlock their best selves, leading powerful sessions that cultivate internal peace, focus, and authentic connection. I strongly believe everyone has the innate ability to heal and transcend. My mission is to make that a reality. Musically, energetically, deeply, and from the heart, I'm dedicated to healing the pain in minds, bodies, and hearts everywhere, bringing people into joyful alignment to share my love for life's infinite possibilities

www.linktr.ee/improvisant

BIG RED AND THE LONG RIDE

by Marissa Shaw

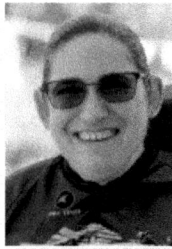

The heat shimmered over Geyserville, California, as a restless breeze danced through the air, carrying the promise of a hot day. It wasn't just any Saturday; it was the day of the Charity Bike Ride, an event that drew cyclists from all over the region to support local initiatives. A palpable energy thrummed through the parking area, a mix of nervous excitement and focused determination. Cyclists milled about, a vibrant kaleidoscope of Lycra and brightly colored helmets, each a whirlwind of last-minute preparations. Helmets were tightened with precise clicks, tires meticulously checked for pressure and wear, and muscles stretched with practiced ease in fluid motions. The mingled scents of sunscreen, the sharp tang of sports rubs, and the sweet, earthy aroma of fresh grapes wafted from the nearby vineyards, creating a uniquely Northern Californian atmosphere, a blend of athletic endeavor and agrarian charm.

Marissa drove her wheelchair beside "Big Red," her striking red recumbent tandem. It wasn't just a bike; it was a statement, a testament to her spirit and her unyielding will. The machine gleamed in the sun. Big Red is a thirty year old bike. Her brakes and gears squeaked when upset, but she moved with determination and spirit, in stark contrast to the younger, lighter recumbent cycles.

Additionally, Big Red represented countless hours of adaptation for Marissa through trial and error, of overcoming physical and societal limitations. She adjusted her padded cushion. She pushed her sunglasses higher on her nose, shielding her eyes from the glare while taking in the scene. Her purple cycling jersey, fitted and comfortable, perfectly matched Big Red's hue, a deliberate choice that echoed her boldness. A long, dark ponytail, symbolizing her strength and resilience, was neatly tucked under her helmet, its weight a familiar comfort, a grounding presence. John, her cycling partner for the first leg, clipped into the front seat, his movements practiced and efficient. John, a longtime friend and fellow cycling enthusiast, had always been one of her biggest supporters, understanding the unique challenges she faced without needing to be told.

"You ready for this?" John asked, turning back with a wide grin. His eyes shone with anticipation, mirroring her excitement but also holding a note of quiet admiration.

Marissa smirked, a flicker of playful defiance in her eyes. "Born ready," she replied, the words echoing a deeper conviction, a mantra she'd repeated to herself countless times in training. In her mind, however, she added, Maybe a little more than ready. I've been waiting for this. This ride was more than just a physical challenge; it was a statement, a rebellion against limitations that others had placed upon her, and that she sometimes even placed upon herself. Growing up with spastic cerebral palsy, Marissa had often been told what she couldn't do. Doctors had painted a picture of restricted mobility, of a life less lived. But Marissa had other plans. Cycling had become her outlet, her way of proving to others and to herself what she was capable of doing. The recumbent tandem, Big Red, was her equalizer, a machine that allowed her to participate fully, without compromise.

Marissa and John had chosen the twenty-seven-mile route, a stretch of road that promised both beauty and challenge, a journey through the heart of wine country. The route snaked past vineyards heavy with ripening grapes, through shaded groves of oak trees, and along stretches of open road where the sun beat down with relentless intensity. The plan was simple: John would pilot Big Red to the pit stop at mile twelve, and then Morgan, with her quiet strength and unwavering support, would guide her the rest of the way. Morgan, a physical therapist by training, had not only helped Marissa with her physical fitness but also her mental fortitude, instilling a belief that went beyond the physical realm. It was a plan carefully laid, like a well-organized map, but Marissa knew plans could shift, just like life itself. She was prepared for the unexpected, for the curveballs that life inevitably threw.

The starting horn blared, a sharp, decisive sound that cut through the morning air, and they were off. The crowd surged forward, a wave of cyclists pedaling with a shared purpose. Marissa felt a surge of adrenaline, the nervous energy now focused into pure determination. This is it, she thought, time to show everyone what you're capable of— time to show herself, too.

The first few miles were a gentle dance along quiet roads, the landscape a tapestry of vineyard rows and sun-kissed hills. The morning sun painted the vines in shades of gold and green, and the air was alive with the hum of insects and the distant call of birds. Marissa leaned into the rhythm of the ride, her legs moving in perfect synchronicity with John's. Big Red glided like a red arrow down the sun-washed road, a seamless, elegant motion that felt almost effortless. The wind whispered past her ears, carrying the scent of wildflowers and damp earth, a heady mix that filled her lungs with each breath. We're doing it, she thought with a surge of pride, just like we practiced. Months of training, early morning rides, and grueling workouts were now paying off.

Along the way, families lined the roads, their faces alight with encouragement. Children held colorful signs that proclaimed "GO RIDERS!" and their small hands waved enthusiastically. Their cheers, though meant for everyone, felt personal, like a special acknowledgment. The sidewalks were a canvas of chalk art, vibrant messages, and drawings of bicycles, creating a festive atmosphere. Some riders zipped past, their eyes darting curiously towards the recumbent tandem. She heard murmurs, "Is that a...?" and caught snippets of conversations. Let them look, she thought. Let them wonder. It fueled her, reminding her of why she was here. Most tandems weren't recumbent, and most riders weren't Marissa. That was the point.

At mile five, they faced their first real climb. The road tilted upwards, and the incline was a slow, steady challenge. The easy rhythm faltered slightly, giving way to a concerted push. John grunted with the exertion, his breath coming in short, sharp bursts. Marissa gritted her teeth, pushing harder, drawing on a reservoir of inner strength, a wellspring of resilience she had cultivated over years of overcoming obstacles. Just breathe, she told herself. You've climbed more challenging hills than this one. She felt the strain in her muscles, the burning sensation in her thighs, but she pushed through, the rhythm of her breathing becoming a steady chant of determination, a silent mantra to keep her going.

"Still with me?" John called, his voice slightly strained.

"Don't make me carry you," she joked back, the familiar banter lightly laced with a steely resolve.

Together, they crested the hill, and the world opened before them. A vast landscape of fields stretched out beneath the azure sky, lavender hills in the distance, and the sun glinting off a distant lake. The view was breathtaking, a moment of tranquility amidst the physical exertion. But Marissa's mind was elsewhere, a memory tugging at the edges of her consciousness.

Something unsettled her. It wasn't just the challenging terrain or the glaring sun. It was a memory, an old ghost that rose whenever she pushed herself too hard, a reminder of vulnerability. She saw herself at thirteen, astride a powerful, unpredictable horse named Danny. He had been tall, fast, and easily spooked, a creature of pure, untamed energy. He was beautiful, she thought, a pang of nostalgia mixed with a touch of fear. On that day, Danny had bolted, his panic a raw, uncontrollable energy. Marissa had held on as long as she could, her small hands gripping the reins, but it hadn't been enough. She had hit the ground hard, the world spinning, and her instructor rushing towards her, face etched with fear and frustration. The fall had left her shaken, bruised, both physically and emotionally, but it hadn't broken her.

Marissa had stood up slowly, her knees trembling, but her eyes filled with sadness. "You okay?" her instructor had asked, voice thick with concern. She had nodded, but her reply was firm: "I don't want to get back on." Shirley, the instructor yelled and said, "Marissa, get back on that horse right now! To move through your fears, you have to face them head on." Marissa got back on the horse with physical assistance, along with grit and determination. That same willpower pulsed through her now, a relentless drive that pushed her forward despite the discomfort and the doubt.

At mile ten, a brown Labrador darted out of a driveway, a flash of fur and an abrupt intrusion into their rhythm. John swerved sharply, narrowly avoiding the dog, the bike wobbling precariously. Marissa's heart leaped into her throat, fear a sudden, icy grip. Hold on, she told herself, just hold on. Then John steadied them, his hands firm on the handlebars.

"You good?" he gasped, his breathing ragged.

She nodded, but her grip tightened on the frame. Too close, she thought, the adrenaline still coursing through her veins. Much too close.

They arrived at the pit stop just after 10:30 AM. Volunteers offered water and snacks, their cheerful encouragement a welcome respite. John dismounted, breathing hard, his face flushed. "Good luck on the next leg" he panted, wiping sweat from his brow.

Marissa gave him a quick, genuine hug. "You did great," she said, and she meant it. She thought, gratitude filling her. "Thank you."
Morgan approached, already in her gear, a confident glint in her eyes. "Ready to rock?" she asked, her voice steady and reassuring.

Marissa took a swig of electrolytes, and the cool liquid was a welcome relief. "Let's go," she said, the words carrying more than just a readiness to continue. It was a declaration. Let's show them what we can do.

The next segment of the ride was tougher. The roads narrowed, winding through less populated areas, and the number of spectators dwindled. Morgan was strong and confident, and she effortlessly kept pace with Marissa. They passed several cyclists struggling on the gradual incline, their faces strained with exertion. Keep going, she thought, sending a boost of encouragement to each rider. You can do this.

Then, mile nineteen.

An orange flag is always mounted on the back of Big Red so motorists and others can see the bike. Morgan and Marissa were at a nice cruising speed when a pickup truck roared down the narrow road beside them. Its music blaring, windows open, the driver oblivious to the cyclists. "Tricycle on your right," someone yelled, the warning sharp and urgent. The truck swerved too close, its wind scared Marissa. Big Red's right rear wheel hit loose gravel, and Morgan fought to keep control to avoid an accident.

A few minutes later as the two were ascending another hill, Big Red came to a screeching halt. The two chains on the bike became entangled in a mess of metal.

Morgan looked at the chains and tried to fix them, but her fingers were too thick to get a proper grip on them.

Not again, her mind screamed, the memory of Danny flooding back with terrifying clarity.

Cyclists quickly gathered around them, their faces concerned. A volunteer radioed for assistance. Marissa sat up slowly, her knees throbbing. A volunteer tried to help her stand. "You should pull yourself out," someone said gently. "You've done enough."

Marissa looked at the bike, with a tear in her eye, and remembered that in the back pouch of Big Red was a number two pencil and some spare chain links. Morgan used the tip of the pencil to gently maneuver the chains apart. The chains were intact except for two small segments that needed to be replaced. Marissa had the parts, and Morgan fixed Big Red. Marissa shook her head. "We're finishing."

Morgan hesitated, then nodded.

By mile twenty-five, every muscle in Marissa's body screamed. An old injury in her knee was acting up, and her legs twitched uncontrollably. But she kept pedaling.

"Almost there!" Morgan called.

The final stretch was uphill. Spectators lined the road, clapping, ringing cowbells.

Marissa's vision blurred. Not from pain, but from something deeper. Something brighter.

Then they crossed the finish line.

Volunteers rushed over with water bottles. Cameras flashed. Someone said, "You're amazing! How do you do it?"

Marissa smiled. But she didn't answer.

Later, under the shade of a massive oak tree, she unstrapped her leg braces and laid back in the grass. Her legs trembled slightly as she stretched them out.

She thought about all the years of being told what she couldn't do. Of falling. Of fighting. Of rising.

No one expected all of these wonderful achievements of a child born with spastic cerebral palsy.

She leaned back, eyes closed, sun warm on her face. She didn't just finish a bike ride.

She proved she could cycle a tough course. She closed her eyes and savored the silence for a moment, a small, well-earned victory. At that moment, Marissa realised she was an athlete.

BIO:

Marissa Shaw is a multi-best-selling co-author and dedicated advocate with over 30 years of experience championing the rights of seniors and people with disabilities. With a Master's degree in Public Administration, Marissa draws from her life experiences with a disability to write compelling, honest narratives that challenge societal norms. Marissa has a deep love for adaptive sports; her chapter in this anthology reflects her passion for cycling and some of her experiences riding her recumbent tandem, affectionately known as Big Red. For any questions regarding adaptive sports, please feel free to contact Marissa.

www.linkedin.com/in/marissa-shaw
www.mobilitymentor.com

ADHD, LYME DISEASE, AND AN AI-LIT PATH

by Rachael Leventhal Garnett

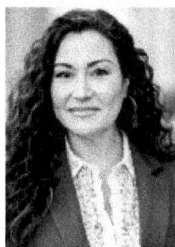

They say, "When life gives you lemons, make lemonade." I've heard that phrase a hundred times, maybe more. Lately, it's been rumbling around my mind. What does it really take to make something sweet out of something sour? You don't just snap your fingers and have lemonade. You need to know how to make it. You need tools. A knife to slice the bitterness open. Water to dilute it. Sugar to soften the tart. A pitcher to hold it all. A spoon (or chopstick) to stir it together.

And time. Time to look for the sugar. Time to remember what you were doing before you opened the fridge and forgot why you were there. Time to read about the history of citrus farming or reorganize the pantry.

So when people say it's simple, like turning struggle into something meaningful, should be fast or easy, I want to say, "*It takes a minute.*"

It's not that I don't want to make lemonade. I'm probably trying to find where the hell I put the knife.

Even when I've had what I needed, actually reading and following the steps has never come naturally. I've always been more spiral than straight. More feel than thought. But I've always had a way of framing things that kept me moving: a dogged optimism, knowing there was something sweeter on the other side. It's a stick-to-itiveness—the desire for action and to try again.

Growing up, I was the girl who didn't fit. Not in elementary school, where I talked too much, fidgeted constantly, and daydreamed while teachers handed me unsatisfactory citizenship grades. Not at the prestigious Hockaday School, where I was clearly not "Hockaday material." And definitely not in the eyes of the college advisor who told me, "Don't bother applying to NYU. They won't want someone like you." I didn't know any better. I thought maybe they were right.

While my classmates breezed through calculus and AP everything, I was shuffled into a new class created just for me, "remedial" math. Bleh... They built resumes, I built secrets. Ones where methamphetamine and cocaine became my misguided coping mechanisms. Yes, they offered an escape, and I had much fun. But they also helped me slow my feral mind.

During my addiction, there was always a flicker in me, a voice that said, "*This is not the end of your story.*" At 28, I made my first big choice. My first decisive transformation. And then came sobriety. Then motherhood. With them, a new resolve: "*Finish what you started.*" I went back to college. First a BFA, then an MA. Willing myself to focus, as if discipline alone could make my mind behave (because nothing says "master of discipline" like Googling how to fold a fitted sheet instead of writing a paper).

Lectures melted into the "wah-wah" of Charlie Brown's teacher's drone. Assignments that took my classmates hours swallowed my days. I'd stare at a syllabus like it was written in a cipher, wondering: *"Why is everything so hard for me? Why am I so bad at life?"* In my wake were unused color-coded planners, unread self-help books, and discarded to-do lists I never looked at.

It wasn't laziness. It wasn't a lack of desire. It was simply a brain wired to see infinite patterns and fantastical possibilities. I could juggle a hundred thoughts at once or zero in so deeply on one idea that the rest of the world disappeared. In museums, I could lose myself for hours, enthralled by Jacob Lawrence's bold narratives of migration or absorbing Ben Shahn's searing social commentaries. But confine me to a lecture hall? No matter how much I loved the art, my mind rebelled like Shahn's protesters pushing against invisible bars. The inability to sit still was also the call to keep moving toward something more alive.

In my mid-30s, I learned the truth. I wasn't broken. I didn't know the recipe that was written for my brain—ADHD, dysgraphia. The diagnoses didn't change who I was. These weren't excuses. They were explanations. They helped me understand the *why*. And I know what a gift that knowledge is. Not everyone gets that clarity.

As humans, we look for meaning. Especially with ADHD, the mind is always in motion, trying to connect, interpret, and understand. Hindsight let me look back and see the shape of things. However, cognitive framing allowed me to hold my past experiences differently as evidence that I adapted the best way I knew how. And that's how I began a new choosing. I gave the past a beloved place in my larger story and allowed myself to embrace a future that honored my spark, accepted the mess, and found sweetness, even when the lemons were sharp.

And then (heavenly music in the background) ... I found estate sales, where history lived in the nicks of rolling pins, not on gallery walls. Because I typically leap without foresight, I didn't know this choice was a giant step into a world where my neurodivergence was an asset. But with a shove from the Divine and a heart that said, *"Yes,"* I chose to thrive on my terms. I'd spent most of my life adapting to systems that weren't built for me. This was one of the first places where I built my own systems, and the world moved with me.

Crowded homes thick with memory, bursting at the seams with lifetimes of accumulation, didn't overwhelm me. They energized me. Here, my brain finally made sense. Hyperfocus turned cluttered home inventories into beautifully curated collections. Intuitive thinking and a knack for spotting what others missed helped me uncover hidden gems in dirty storage buildings. The restless, relentless creativity and the boundless ADHD energy fueled it all.

Neurodivergence was my superpower in a world of fragmented multi-tasks and unpredictable discoveries. For the first time, I felt successful, confident, and truly me. My estate sale business flourished because of my ADHD. All the things I once thought made me bad at life turned out to be what made me great in this career. My brain and I were on the same team. I was living my version of happily ever after.

Until a tiny, uninvited guest rewired my nervous system.

I don't remember when I got the tick bite. I remember the bullseye rash and never thought of it again after it faded. For years, I blamed mounting fatigue and joint pain on burnout. Of course, my body ached. I was a mother of two active boys running a business powered by hyperactivity, black coffee, and an alarming amount of candy. The brain fog? Just the tax of a mind that never stopped spinning. Losing track of conversation mid-sentence? *"Classic executive dysfunction,"* I told myself. Forgetting my phone number. That was something else entirely. But I'd spent a lifetime compensating for a restless brain; I thought these were more hurdles to outmaneuver.

But then the ground shifted. It started with the words dissolving on my tongue like sugar in the rain. I'd reach for *"umbrella"* and grasp at *"that thing… the sky-cover?"* My hands, once deft at untangling necklace knots or keying numbers on a cash register, stiffened and ached, my knuckles twisting with nodule growths until turning a doorknob became a struggle. The fatigue wasn't the familiar crash after a marathon of productivity; it was a lead blanket.

My superpowers disappeared. The hyperfocus that once let me spot the 1st edition, seven-volume set of Charles F. Haanel's *Master Key System* in a mountain of books? Gone. The lightning-fast ability to make connections, the spontaneous problem-solving, the joyful obsessiveness, the intuitive leaps, and the vivaciousness were also gone. It was like someone unplugged me.

The tiny spirochete *Borrelia burgdorferi*, the culprit in Lyme disease, doesn't just attack joints or cause rashes. It's a saboteur of the nervous system, slipping past the blood-brain barrier to rewire cognition. For someone already navigating ADHD, the overlap is a cruel magic trick. It wasn't just "brain fog"—it was inflammation disrupting neural pathways, making even simple words dissolve on my tongue. And the crushing fatigue was mitochondrial dysfunction, cells starving for energy. And that alarming amount of candy I'd lived on for years? Pure fuel for Lyme disease.

For eight months, I lived only in my bedroom, except for a long stint in the hospital. Doctors threw ridiculous guesses like darts: *Flu. Meningitis. Hepatitis C. Liver cancer.* Each test came back negative. "We don't know what's wrong with you." The not-knowing was its own kind of torture. At least a label is an enemy you can learn to fight. But how do you wage war on a ghost?

I lost months with my boys. Their voices, once the compass of my days, faded into a fog I couldn't penetrate. "Mom's just tired," they were told. But being exhausted doesn't make you forget your child's middle name. Tired doesn't make you pray, fists clenched in the dark, *"Let me not wake up."*

The business I'd built, the one that made ADHD my greatest gift, collapsed. There was no grand finale, no carefully curated last sale—just silence, a voicemail full of confused employees, and the sour taste of surrender.

There's a special loneliness in being told you're dying, then almost immediately being told you're not, multiple times. But feeling your body rot from the inside. It was my father, a retired surgeon, who made the diagnosis.

"Baby," he said over the phone, "you have Lyme disease."

And then—the aha moment! The memory of the bullseye rash I'd shown my husband and shrugged off. Lyme disease had been etching its signature into me for years.

The ADHD diagnosis felt like a door opening. But when the illness is chronic and late-stage, the door leads to a battlefield, not a cure. The relief of knowing collided with the grief of *too late*. The spirochetes had already tunneled into my nervous system, rewriting my chemistry. ADHD was now tangled with Lyme disease's neurological sabotage. The focus, energy, and my very self had been hijacked.

I threw myself into a functional medicine protocol: supplements, herbs, infrared saunas, dietary overhauls, each tiny step, disbelief that this was forever. But healing is a spiral. Some days, I climbed; some weeks, I slid back into Lymey exhaustion and mush.

When I was finally strong enough to work again, I faced a cruel truth: the life I'd loved wouldn't fit this changed body and mind. Estate sales demanded a physicality I no longer had: the lifting, the hauling, the marathon days digging through garages in the Texas heat. I mourned it like a death. That business was proof that I wasn't flawed; it was the lens that let me see treasure in myself where others saw trash.

So, I did what defeated survivors do: grieve, struggle, and cope. Out of tremendous guilt and what I saw as failure, I took what I thought I deserved: the dreaded desk job, stale office air, fluorescent lights, and a paycheck that didn't cover my bills. The voice in my head whispered, harsh as ever, *"This is what you're worth now."*

I didn't pivot. Not right away. For a long time, I felt like a shell of the person I'd been—exhausted, flattened, and shrunken. I worked for people who didn't see me, didn't value me, and somewhere in the weight of that dismissal, I lost my voice. My power. I moved through a life that didn't fit, wearing a version of myself that didn't feel like mine.

And then, in the doldrums of the life I didn't want, I started playing with AI-assisted art.

I needed something low-stakes and creative, a place to experiment without lifting boxes or pretending I had the energy to push through. I needed something that didn't care if I couldn't finish.

At first, it was just curiosity. I messed around with the earliest text-to-image AI art generators, typing in odd little prompts and seeing what came out. Cowboy cats made of wood. Felt cats in magnetic storms. Whimsical, melancholic, and utterly alive, like my brain turned inside out and offered to me as proof I still existed.

Looking back, it was the medicine I didn't know I needed. I wasn't speaking or writing in the usual sense; I was imagining and telling visual stories.

It turns out that matters.

Lyme disease mimics dementia on some days and ADHD on others, leaving you unsure which part of your brain you've lost and which you're still holding on to.

I didn't know it then, but research shows that creative language, such as metaphor, storytelling, and visual imagery, lights up different parts of the brain than everyday communication does. Neuroinflammation blocks the usual routes, but creativity can take the back roads.

When I talked or tried to write something practical, an email, a message, a simple explanation, I'd lose my place, mid-thought. But when I used words to make art to shape an image, I didn't lose the thread. The thinking held and the words stayed. That was wild. It felt like my brain had found a side door, and for once, it let me all the way through.

I didn't have even an iota that this little hobby would become the scaffolding holding my fractured cognition together. The same attention to detail that once helped me find a bar of gold in a washing machine (yes, a big bar of gold) now laser-targeted the perfect word sequence to create a world of anthropomorphic AI cats. Each image I generated whispered the same message: *"I am still here."*

Then, ChatGPT came along. Around the same time, my short-term memory and language retrieval were still shot. I'd stare at blank emails, struggling to remember words as basic as *"reschedule"* or *"apologize."* I typed whatever fragments I had, half-thoughts and hints towards meaning, and ChatGPT filled in the blanks.

What surprised me was how I began to feel. The dread I carried into every writing task began to lift. Something or someone was there with me, and I started showing up differently—calmer, clearer, less afraid of forgetting, and less ashamed.

As much as I love AI. It didn't fix me. I made the choice. Slowly, I started reclaiming space: meditation, affirmations on my vanity mirror, and music that reminded me, *"I'm badass."* I unfollowed and unsubscribed from the people and things that no longer served my highest good. I reconnected with the Source of Light that had always been inside me.

As the dust cleared, something new took root. The more I used AI, the more curious I became about how it worked. I started studying prompts like puzzles, tinkering with phrases, testing combinations, and chasing that moment when it clicked. The output felt like something I thought about but couldn't quite say. I found a lifeline, a language, a ladder.

I didn't set out to become an AI consultant. I was trying to survive my job, function with a broken brain, and find a way to communicate again. But the more I learned, the more I saw what was possible, not just for me, but for others. What started as a coping tool became a calling. I wanted to share what I'd discovered with people like me who were searching for a way through.

Somewhere in the building, the tinkering, the learning, and the sharing, my joy returned. The love of life I thought I'd lost somewhere in a hospital bed and under the weight of too many blank days came back, too. I found my dogged, incurable optimism and the belief that beauty was still ahead. And I found my love for being alive—for mornings that smell like coffee, cats purring on my keyboard, connection, color, and the strange wonder of just being *here*.

I didn't choose ADHD or Lyme disease. One shaped the way I lived in the world. The other tried to stop me altogether. Nudged by something bigger than myself and open enough to say, *"yes,"* I stopped waiting for the recipe to make sense and started slicing the lemons I had.

The damage didn't vanish. ADHD is still here, amplified and mutated by Lyme. I still lose words. Still get foggy. Still retreat from exhaustion. But now, I know how to build around it.

Even now, I'll be in the middle of talking and… poof… the rest of the sentence just disappears. People always say, "You sound great." which is sweet, but they didn't know me before when I was fast, clever, and a little intimidating. These days, I trail off, invent nonsense words, and have learned to laugh at the blanks. It's frustrating, sure, but maybe it's charming? Like I'm sprinkling in dramatic silence on purpose—very avant-garde of me.

But when I use words to make images, they stay. I don't lose them. That's still the strangest and most beautiful thing to me.

I will never have an appreciation for what Lyme disease did to me. It dismantled my life, health, memory, work, and confidence. Even ADHD, once the source of my sparkle, went dim. But it didn't disappear, it adapted. I still hyperfocus. I still get lit up by ideas, fall down glorious rabbit holes, and connect things most people overlook. That's the part of my brain I've always treasured. Now, though, I don't always get to keep the whole shape of the brilliance. Lyme disease makes it harder to hold. Still, I get to decide what that means. I can mourn what was stolen and still find value in what remains. That's the meaning I carry. I can let go of who I was without letting go of who I am. I became someone who knows how to make something from what remains.

Maybe it took so long because the universe held me still until I could find the path to a tool that helped something good grow out of what broke me.

But, I've learned that the tools don't change us. We do. We are the heroes.

Your tool might not be AI. It could be painting, running, golfing, poetry, or prayer. The point was never the tool. It's the choice to find the knife, reach for the sugar, and keep stirring.

Because you are not broken.

You are not behind.

You are not bad at life.

You're just holding lemons, waiting for the recipe to reveal itself. And trust me, there's sweetness in there somewhere. Keep looking.

BIO:

Rachael Leventhal Garnett is a pioneering voice at the intersection of artificial intelligence and human connection. With a background spanning visual art, estate sales, and hypnotherapy, she sees connections others often miss. A three-time bestselling co-author, educator, speaker, and AI-assisted artist, she helps people navigate rapid change with clarity and confidence.

As co-founder of EaaS AI and one of the first AI-certified consultants globally, Rachael trains teams to integrate AI in ways that are strategic, intuitive, and deeply human. Through workshops, panels, one-on-one consulting, and podcast conversations, she helps organizations move from overwhelm to action, translating uncertainty into practical, grounded innovation. Whether it's streamlining workflows or building custom GPTs, her focus is always on making AI work for real people in the real world.

Her work is rooted in a simple belief: that the most powerful evolution happens at the intersection of human insight and intelligent tools. She speaks nationwide and partners with mission-driven organizations to make AI accessible, meaningful, and usable.

Married for twenty-six years to her favorite person, Matthew, Rachael has two fabulous adult sons and a clowder of opinionated cats. Online, she's known as the LinkedIn Cat Lady, a title she wears proudly.
An incurable optimist, she believes we're not broken, we're just waiting for the right tools, the right timing, and the right story to remind us of what we already know.

lp.eaaservice.com/Top10

www.linkedin.com/in/rachael-garnett-eaas

THE STORM THAT SPARKED MY LIGHT

by Sandra Bothe

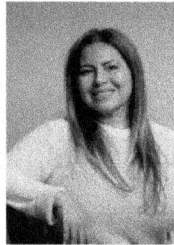

Before I Knew ADHD

The first note from Zach's kindergarten teacher, Ms. Moskowitz, came home in Zach's backpack. It was folded neatly, tucked between drawings of trees and rockets. I unfolded it casually, expecting another reminder about lunch boxes or reading logs.

Instead, it read:

"Zach is having difficulty staying in his seat. He gets up often, talks during instruction, and struggles to follow directions."

I blinked.

He was five.

How could anyone expect a five-year-old boy to sit still all day?

I brushed it off, politely but internally annoyed. I told myself, "The problem isn't Zach; it's a classroom trying to train children into stillness."

After all, my son was bright. Curious. Energetic.

Of course, he moved around.

Of course, he talked when he had a thought. What five-year-old doesn't?

But then came another note. And another.

Different words, same message.

I started to feel like I was being told something about my child that I didn't want to hear.

And still, I didn't think of it as a problem.

I thought of it as personality.

When the World Shut Down, My Eyes Began to Open

Then COVID hit.

The classroom disappeared.

The backpack stayed hung.

And suddenly, school lived inside our house and inside my laptop screen.

I watched Zach try to sit through remote lessons on the living room couch.

One minute, he was present. Focused.

The next, he was upside down, his feet on the cushions, his eyes somewhere far away.

"Zach, pay attention," I'd whisper from across the room.

"Zach, the teacher's talking."

"Zach, what did she just say?"

But his mind had already sprinted three miles ahead.

Not distracted... just elsewhere.

Every ten minutes felt like an hour.

The fidgeting. The humming. The constant need for movement.

The way he'd interrupt, not out of rudeness, but urgency, like he'd burst if he didn't speak immediately.

At first, I told myself: it's the pandemic. Everyone's struggling.

But by the end of first grade, something in me began to shift.

Because watching him... I started to see myself.

Second Grade, Second Glance

When in-person school resumed, I hoped things would smooth out.

He'd have structure. A teacher. Classmates. A routine.

But halfway into second grade, another meeting. Another teacher.

Another version of the same sentence:

"Zach is a bright, sweet kid. But he has trouble staying on task. He zones out. He gets up. He talks over others."

This time, I didn't brush it off.

This time, the words landed deeper.

I was concerned about him because they sounded painfully familiar, and it was the first time they had sounded this familiar.

It was like someone had cracked open a time capsule.

Because I remembered the girl who couldn't finish a task unless it was on a deadline.

The girl who reread the same paragraph five times, got distracted in the middle of it, and didn't remember what it said.

The one who was praised for being helpful, agreeable, and quiet.

But inside, I was endlessly restless.

That's when I started reading about ADHD.

And somewhere between the checklists and case studies, a strange kind of grief washed over me.

Grief for not knowing sooner.

Grief for how hard I had worked to keep up.

Grief for the version of me without any idea why everything always felt harder, louder, faster.

That was the day I stopped seeing ADHD as his story.

I started understanding it as part of mine, too.

The Quiet Storm

As a little girl, I didn't bounce off walls.

I bounced inside my head.

My body stayed still, but my mind? It was always moving, scanning, skipping, rehearsing, imagining, fixing, planning, overthinking, editing.

I could sit through hours of school without saying much. But inside, it was chaos.

The adults around me thought I was a dream student; quiet, polite, and adaptable.

And I was. I had learned early that being easy to deal with made people happy.

I smiled when I was supposed to.

I followed the rules, helped at home, and said thank you even when my insides screamed, "This isn't fair."

If there was a problem, I solved it.

If someone was upset, I tried to make it better.

No one saw the part of me that couldn't sit through a full homework assignment without standing up for a snack, then a drink, and then remembering I had to organize my pencils.

No one saw the frustration I carried quietly when my mind would jump ahead too fast, skip a step, or forget the question by the time I got to it.

I didn't have tantrums.

I had mental replays of everything I could have done better.

I didn't get detention.

I gave myself a private punishment of shame and silence.

When I was overwhelmed, I didn't lash out.

I became invisible.

I didn't know I was masking. I just thought I was doing what I needed to survive.

To be liked.

To be good.

It turns out many girls with ADHD do precisely that.

They internalize. They comply. They overachieve and then crash.

And because they don't cause problems, they often go unnoticed for years.

That was me.

The Hidden Cost of Coping

I didn't know that coping had a cost.

I thought I was strong because I could keep going. I didn't complain. I got good grades. I held jobs. I smiled in public and carried my storms in silence.

But over time, the mask became heavy.

Not just emotionally but physically.

There were days when I felt like I was moving through life in overdrive, hyper-aware, always thinking, always preparing, always anticipating what might go wrong to stay one step ahead.

I didn't forget what I was doing.

I remembered everything, the deadlines, the details, the conversations from days ago.

And that was part of the exhaustion.

Because my mind never let go.

I blamed stress. Work. Life.

But I didn't see that constantly operating on high alert wasn't resilience, it was depletion.

It was anxiety dressed up as responsibility.

It was self-abandonment masked as competence.

Every unchecked pressure quietly compounded until I couldn't distinguish between doing my best and running on fumes.

And what I wish someone had told me sooner was this:

Coping is not the same as thriving.

High-functioning is not the same as being well.

Because when you're constantly scanning, pleasing, and fixing, you lose the ability to ask yourself: What do I need?

That realization didn't just open my eyes.

It opened the door to self-compassion I didn't know I'd been locked out of.

Thriving (and Hiding) in a Corporate Life

When I landed my first corporate job in my twenties, I felt like I had arrived.

The pace was fast. The work was demanding. Every day brought a new challenge.

And me? I thrived.

My to-do list was never short, and my calendar looked like a game of Tetris. I was the go-to person when something needed to get done fast. Tight deadlines, unexpected problems, juggling five things at once? I was in my element.

People praised me for being driven and high-energy.

But they didn't see the engine behind it all, a brain that had to stay in motion.

Slowness felt like suffocation.

Routine felt like a trap.

What looked like efficiency was actually urgency.

I wasn't working a lot because I was organized.

I was working a lot because my brain didn't know how to slow down.

And in the early years, it worked.

Though I didn't know it then, ADHD gave me strengths that fit the chaos of logistics and operations.

I could spot patterns quickly, shift tasks midstream, and jump into problems without needing all the information.

I was intuitive, fast, and resourceful.

A storm with purpose.

But the higher I climbed, the more the ground changed.

Less doing, more planning.

Less reacting, more structure.

And when I finally did focus, I couldn't stop.

I was drowning.

I would spend entire days answering emails, unable to stop because each message felt like a puzzle, and puzzles are challenging to walk away from when you have a brain that thrives on novelty.

People around me could pause their inboxes and focus on one thing at a time.

I couldn't.

Every ping pulled my attention.

Every quick question led to ten others.

I'd stay late catching up on the actual work, exhausted, frustrated, and confused about why I couldn't keep up.

It was like trying to row a boat with no oars, just instinct and adrenaline.

The same traits that once felt like my superpower were now burning me out.

And I blamed myself.

I thought I was just not focused enough. I always felt the urge to do five tasks at the same time. I was running a race with weights on my ankles and still finishing the lap.

And I just thought I had to try harder.

From Denial to Discovery

I didn't go looking for a diagnosis.

I went looking for a way to help my son.

After that second-grade meeting, I did what any mother would do: I started reading, Googling, Watching YouTube videos, and downloading parenting books with titles like Raising a Child with ADHD.

At first, I kept a healthy distance.

This is for Zach, I reminded myself.

Not for me.

But the deeper I went, the harder that line became to hold.

The descriptions didn't just fit my son.

They described me perfectly.

- Difficulty starting tasks unless they are urgent.

- Racing thoughts.

- Trouble listening when my mind was already ahead.

- Feeling overwhelmed by small decisions.

- Thriving in chaos but wilting in structure.

I wasn't just reading about him.

I was reading about me, the version of me I had hidden, adapted, and masked for decades.

And suddenly, memories came flooding back:

- I started the high school assignments the day before they were due.

- The shame I carried every time I was distracted despite trying so hard to stay focused.

It all started making sense.

ADHD, or Attention Deficit Hyperactivity Disorder, is a neurodevelopmental condition that affects how the brain manages attention, energy, and executive function, like task initiation, emotional regulation, and prioritization. It doesn't look the same for everyone.

While the classic image often involves physical hyperactivity, many adults, especially women, present differently.

We're often organized, reliable, and high achieving on the outside while privately battling mental restlessness, overstimulation, and a deep sense of overwhelm.

I always had a strong memory and followed through with my responsibilities. In fact, I was often praised for my attention to detail. But I needed urgency to stay engaged. I overthought small decisions. I'd go from task to task because my brain craved stimulation.

What I've come to understand is that ADHD doesn't cancel out your strengths; it just adds extra layers to how you manage them. Many develop high-functioning coping strategies that help them perform until they burn out.

And for decades, because I didn't match the stereotype, I never imagined ADHD could be part of my story.

But it is.

Now that I know, I finally have the language to understand myself with clarity and compassion.

And then I read this:

"ADHD in women often goes undiagnosed because it looks different. Instead of disruption, it shows up as internal chaos, perfectionism, and emotional overwhelm, often misinterpreted as personality flaws."

— Journal of Clinical Child and Adolescent Psychology

I paused.

I reread it.

Internal chaos. Perfectionism. Emotional overwhelm.

It was like someone had turned on the lights in a room I didn't even know I was living in.

I wasn't weak.

I wasn't broken.

I was neurodivergent.

And the diagnosis I had feared, if I'm honest, brought something unexpected.

Relief.

It was a quiet, surprising kind of relief that whispered, "It's not your fault. You are just wired differently." And you did the best you could with no manual.

Home Life Understood, Not Judged

Looking back, I realized how many moments at home were shaped by a brain that wouldn't slow down and a heart that didn't know why.

I wasn't trying to be complicated.

I wasn't trying to dominate conversations or interrupt.

But the thoughts came fast; if I didn't say them aloud, they'd disappear.

In the middle of my husband's story, I'd jump in, not to cut him off but because I was excited, or I made a connection, or I suddenly remembered something from two days ago that felt urgent in that exact second.

He'd get frustrated.

Rightfully so.

He'd say, "Please let me finish."

And I'd shrink.

Not because I didn't care.

But because I didn't know how often I did it.

I'd feel ashamed. And then I'd get defensive.

Which turned into tension. Distance. Misunderstanding.

Before I knew I had ADHD, I thought this was a personality flaw.

I thought I just needed to be better. Listen more. Try harder.

And I did try. But it always felt like I was swimming against the current.

After I started understanding ADHD, I began to understand myself.

And when I shared what I was learning with my husband, something shifted for both of us.

He stopped taking my interruptions so personally.

I started becoming more aware of them.

We added tools, small things that made a big difference.

I'd write things down instead of blurting them out.

He'd gently remind me when I spiraled into too many tabs, mentally or literally.

The most significant shift wasn't tactical.

It was emotional.

We moved from judgment to compassion.

From "Why are you like this?" to "How can I support you?"

From silence to understanding.

We learned how to dance with the rhythm of my mind instead of fighting it.

It wasn't perfect.

But it was real.

Breaking the Mold for My Son

If there's one thing harder than living with undiagnosed ADHD, it's watching your child face the same challenges and be misunderstood the same way.

By the time Zach returned to school in second grade, I had a deeper awareness.

But the system hadn't changed.

It was still built around stillness, sameness, and silence.

None of which matched the way his brain, or mine, worked.

I remember one day in particular.

He came home quietly. Head down.

His teacher had made him stay in the corner of the classroom because he "couldn't stay in his seat."

He was seven.

Seven.

I could feel my anger rising, not toward the teacher; she wasn't cruel. She was doing her best with the tools she had.

But I realized that those tools weren't made for kids like Zach.

I saw how the school expected him to learn in one way: sit, listen, repeat.

But his brain? It needed movement.

It needed interest, urgency, and interaction.

He wasn't misbehaving. He was coping.

Until then, advocacy wasn't something I used to do.

But I discovered I needed to speak up for my son.

So, I started asking for meetings.

I shared what I was learning about ADHD, not just from articles but from experience.

I explained that the movement wasn't defiance; it was regulation.

That interruption wasn't rudeness but timing issues in a brain wired for speed.

I also made changes at home.

We used visual schedules.

I offered movement breaks before and after homework.

We added timers and chunked tasks into bite-size pieces.

I stopped punishing him for things I now understood he couldn't fully control.

And most of all, I reminded him:

"You're not broken. You're brilliant. You just learn differently. And that's okay."

The more I unlearned the expectations that had once weighed me down, the more I could free him from them.

I wasn't just parenting my son.

I was reparenting myself.

A New Legacy

Zach doesn't need to be like everyone else.

And neither do I.

That's the legacy I want to leave, not one of silent struggle but of bold self-acceptance.

He doesn't have to earn his worth by overachieving or proving he can "behave."

He is worthy precisely as he is, curious, intense, full of light.

And as his mother, my most significant task is not to fix him.

It's to see him.

To give him language for what he feels.

To teach him that regulation is a skill, not a character flaw.

To show him by example, growth begins when we stop hiding who we are.

Because the world doesn't need more perfect children.

It needs more kids who are allowed to be human—messy, vibrant, wiggly, and wonderfully unique.

And as I raise him with new tools, I'm also raising the younger version of myself who didn't have them.

We are building a new rhythm together. One where differences are not just accepted but embraced.

If I can help him meet himself with compassion earlier than I did,

then every challenging moment, every misunderstood year, and every quiet shame I carried, will have paved the way for something greater.

A new legacy.

One rooted not in conformity but in truth.

Reframing ADHD: Not Broken, Just Wired Differently

There was a time when I thought ADHD was something to fix.

A problem to solve.

A label to avoid.

Now, I see it differently.

ADHD isn't a flaw.

It's a different operating system.

Like any system, it needs the right environment, the right tools, and, most of all, the right understanding.

I used to beat myself up for being unable to focus like others.

Now I know: I can focus intensely when something matters, when it's urgent, or when it sparks interest.

That's not a failure. That's how my brain works.

We're not driven by importance. We're driven by engagement.

I've also learned to work with my brain, not against it.

- Setting time blocks during my day to give my mind structure and rhythm.

- I prioritize by energy, not just urgency, so I don't burn out on the wrong things.

- I keep visual reminders around me because out of sight truly means out of mind.

But the most significant shift wasn't about tools.

It was about permission.

Permission to stop shaming myself.

To stop calling myself scattered and inconsistent.

I want to see my creativity, passion, and intensity for what they really are: gifts.

Embracing my ADHD didn't hold me back, it awakened me.

My brain wasn't broken; it was built for creativity, connection, and reinvention.

I needed to run free to pursue what I'm passionate about.

Once I stopped trying to fit into expectations that didn't match how I naturally operate, I began to dedicate time beyond my job to learn what truly lit me up: mindset, the unconscious mind, communication, and language.

That path led me to Neuro-Linguistic Programming (NLP), where I became a certified coach, and for the first time, I understood myself on a whole new level. I found why it was so difficult to always use my voice, in any room, to embrace self- expression with confidence.

Then came Mental Emotional Release and Hypnotherapy, where I rewired the beliefs that had held me back for years.

And through HUNA, spirituality, energy, and meditation, I found a deeper inner peace and presence. It became the soul of my transformation.

This isn't just a passion anymore, it is a calling.

I launched my own business, started writing my first book, and published it. I have always wanted to write since I was young.

In the process of writing it, I discovered powerful clarity about my purpose.

Then I trained in public speaking, became a Certified NLP Trainer's Trainer, and stepped onto a stage to share my story in front of hundreds.

None of this would have happened, if I hadn't first decided to stop hiding from how my brain was wired, and start building with it instead.

No one is to blame.

I never disclosed what I didn't fully understand.

And truthfully, I didn't feel safe enough to.

So, at the time, I pushed through.

And I burned out, before I found my authentic path.

There were late nights, catching up on tasks, I filled my calendar, answered every message, checked every box for the outside, while the inside felt empty.

I was quietly unraveling inside.

I wasn't tired because I was doing too much.

I was tired because I wasn't investing my time wisely in my passions and the things that mattered to me.

Until I understood I wasn't broken.

I was misaligned.

Misalignment is not a life sentence; it's a redirection.

Understanding ADHD gave me more than insight; it gave me permission to pivot and heal. I want to build something that reflects me, not the version I have performed for years.

I'm building a business that reflects who I am, where my ideas are fuel, not flaws.

Today I'm working on what I love: mindset, spirituality, behavior, transformation, and human potential.

I stopped apologizing for how I process the world.

I'm not chasing perfection. I'm living on purpose.

ADHD didn't take anything from me.

What hurt was not knowing I had it but blaming myself for the symptoms;

feeling guilty for needing more movement, flexibility, and heart in what I do.

In their place, I found pride.

I can generate ideas, connect dots, feel deeply, and lead from the inside out.

My brain didn't fail me.

It saved me.

It led me out of a life that looked perfect on paper and into one that felt purposeful in my soul.

Now I see it for what it is:

A mind that moves like wind, unseen but powerful.

A brain that builds storms and also creates lightning.

A path that's not always straight but leads to surprising places.

Today, I'm not just managing ADHD.

I'm rewriting my story with it.

And in doing so, I hope others can do the same.

We are more than our diagnosis.

We are the authors of our own rewiring.

And when we stop trying to be like everyone else…

We finally discover the extraordinary in how we were made.

BIO:

Sandra Bothe is a first-generation Latina, Founder of Thriving Mindsets, Master Practitioner of Mental Emotional Release® and Hypnotherapy, Trainer of Advanced Neuro-Linguistic Programming, Mindfulness and Transformational Coach.

With nearly two decades of experience as a Global Logistics and Supply Chain corporate leader, her journey through the intricate landscape of Corporate America, as an immigrant, became the catalyst for founding Thriving Mindsets. This visionary organization empowers immigrant professionals and entrepreneurs to silence self-doubt, cultivate confidence, amplify their voices, and boldly step into their power. As a passionate writer and speaker, she uses her voice to champion Inclusion, inspiring others to rise, lead, and thrive.

Writing her debut book, Unmuting Myself—A Voice Silenced by Doubt Dared to Rise, and speaking on stages reflect her unwavering commitment to using her voice in service of a world where everyone feels a true sense of belonging. Through powerful storytelling and cultural insight, she challenges traditional narratives around identity and inclusion, unmuting voices, one courageous story at a time.

www.linkedin.com/in/sandra-bothe

www.amazon.com/dp/B0F6L5WHPB

SHIFT YOUR GAZE AND SEE ME
by Sharon Birn

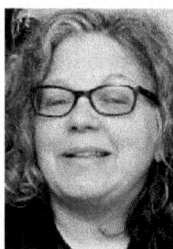

"See Me"

By Sharon Birn

Came two months early, breathin' thin air,
Doctors weren't sure I'd make it from there.
But I fought like a flame that refused to die,
With a will so strong and a fire in my eye.

They gave my folks a list of "can't" and "won't,"
Said there's a lot she just won't own.
But I was born to prove 'em wrong,
And honey, I've been doin' that all along.

So don't just see the chair I ride,
See the girl with grit and dreams inside.
Don't see limits—see the climb,
The mountain I conquer every time.

I ain't the "less" that some folks see,
I'm a whole damn storm of ability.
So if you're lookin'—look deep and free,
Open your heart… and see me.

Yeah, they see the wheels, but they miss the wings,
The strength I've got, the hope it brings.
This chair ain't chains—it sets me free,
Gives me the power to just be me.

They talk about courage like it's a prize,
But I've been living brave all my life.
Don't need your pity, don't need your praise,
Just need the world to shift its gaze.

So don't just see the chair I roll,
See the woman with a burning soul.
Don't see broken—see the fight,
The road I ride, the dreams in sight.
I'm not your burden, not your cause,
I'm a lightning bolt with battle scars.
So if you're starin'—look and see,
There's more to me… now see me.

What if you looked through a different lens,
Where strength comes wrapped in all kinds of skin?
What if you saw me for all I do,
Not just how I move, but what I push through?

I've been told "you can't" more times than I can say.
But I've turned every "no" into a brand-new way.
This life ain't easy, but it's mine to steer—
I rise each day, and I ride without fear.

So don't just see this chair I ride,
See the fire that won't hide.
I was made for more than sympathy—
I'm purpose, power, and legacy.
I ain't your lesson, I ain't your myth,

I'm the proof that strength exists.
So open up your eyes and be—
The kind of soul who sees me.

See me rise…
See me real…
See me whole…
Behind the wheel.
I'm not just rollin'… I'm runnin' free.
Look past the frame…
And see me.

©Sharon Birn 4-19-25

At age 55, I had an epiphany that shocked and liberated me. I realized that while I've spent much of my life pushing beyond the boxes that others tried to fit me into, I was also, unknowingly, pushing my body past its limits to prove I was more than my diagnosis. And while my intention was strength, what I needed—what I deserved—was compassion, especially from myself.

I experience chronic medical conditions that can vary in intensity from day to day. These medical conditions are secondary to my primary diagnosis, a neurological disability, cerebral palsy, CP for short.

This was the very first label /diagnosis I received. At 18 months old, my parents had gotten answers to why all the things that were happening with my little body were occurring, and why developmental milestones weren't being reached. My mother's instinct that something was wrong with me was finally validated. It was one of the validations in her life that she never wanted to receive. On the other hand, she was glad to finally have answers. There was a reason for my struggles, and that reason was Cerebral Palsy (CP).

Finally, people stopped telling my mother that she was a nervous mother who was just comparing her second child to her older sister, that there was nothing wrong with me, and that she needed to stop the comparison game
Something else happened once I got the diagnosis.

They gave my folks a list of "can't" and "won't,"
Said there's a lot she just won't own.

©Sharon Birn 4-19-25

I became boxed in and defined by what my perceived limitations would be because of my diagnosis; developing abilities didn't even enter the conversations. Thankfully, my parents did not buy into the idea that I was a list of "can't" and "won't", and as I grew up, they taught me not to buy into this mindset either. I am beyond grateful for my parents' belief in me and my abilities, despite how frightened they were that they did not know what the future would hold for me, and what if the "experts" were right?

The trend of people seeing my wheelchair and making assumptions about all the things I can't do, or what lights me up with enthusiasm, still happens today. Yes, in 2025, as far as our society has come, there is still a long way to go; it's an interesting phenomenon that still boggles my mind.

I was the first person with a physical disability to be mainstreamed into my public school district in 1979, after the Individuals with Disabilities Education Act (IDEA) was passed. It stated that school districts had to educate students with disabilities in their home districts, where possible and appropriate. I was placed in special education to "help me catch up" to grade level. Also, because of my neurodivergence, another term that was placed upon me by expert professionals, as a way to explain that I learn and process information differently, from those who are neurotypical.

Being the first person mainstreamed into my school district made me known as the girl in the wheelchair who sometimes happened to have the name "Sharon". This trend continued throughout high school.

I have always seen myself, even as a child, as more than my diagnosis, but the world around me did not, and often still does not. When I was younger, it was drilled into me that I had to learn to live with my disability and push beyond obstacles and pain daily. Continuing to function and accomplish my daily responsibilities, no matter what. School work and social engagements had to be kept. As the saying goes, "The show must go on."

This philosophy served me well growing up; the more somebody told me I couldn't do something, the more determined I was to make it happen and prove them wrong. However, every coin has two sides, and the flip side of this coin is the downside.

Pushing to be more than my perceived deficits, which others assigned to me, often meant that I wasn't listening to my body's messages. The messages were trying to alert me that I needed to take a break and take time off to attend to myself. I couldn't do that; I would be seen as a failure, and lesser than because I was playing the victim card.

Pushing myself this way led to years of internal self-defamation and negative self-talk. I bought and recited the narrative of others that I was playing victim and looking for pity. I beat myself up when I could not hide that I was experiencing tremendous levels of pain and frustration.

Beating myself up for exposing my struggles, and allowing myself to be vulnerable in this way, became a pastime for me, like Major League Baseball is considered a National pastime in America.

After many years of self-criticism, pushing myself to be "strong" and function through enormous discomfort and tremendous pain, I eventually realized this did not make me more than my diagnosis, not at all. This realization really shook me; I needed to make a shift. I started leaning into the truth that I had always known. What makes me more than my diagnoses are all of the parts of me, including learning to prioritize listening to my body.

The need to push and push beyond the label was so critical to me because society made judgments about my capabilities, or lack thereof, solely on the fact that I used a wheelchair full-time to get around. Throughout my life, I have had family members, friends, employers, teachers, restaurant employees, and other people who work in social venues, make everything about my cerebral palsy. One example is a teacher I had in high school who told my parents," When I saw her in her wheelchair, I assumed her brain didn't work." However, he realized he was very wrong when I was one of the top students in his class that year.

I have had employers tell me that I was being passed up for a promotion, because they didn't know how to accommodate the position, around the needs of my disability. My spouse divorced me, stating my disability had become more than he could handle, and he wanted to be free to live his life unencumbered. Although I know there was a lot more that contributed to the demise of our marriage, I would be lying if I said those words did not sting and imprint on my soul, for a long time.

I am not someone's burden or cause; I am a valuable, contributing member of my family, community, and society. Every human being needs help with some things. No one can be completely 100% independent when striving to achieve their goals. What differs is not that we need help, but what we need help with.

These things could have led me to crawl into a hole and never come out. If you know me, you know that from when I was very young, I would not have made that choice. Instead, I decided, and I continue to choose, to be more than my diagnoses. I do this, simply, by staying present.

I desire to learn from my past experiences, not live in them. I am very intentional about writing my story. I no longer allow myself to live by other people's narratives. I require myself to show up unapologetically and authentically everywhere I go.

Having Cerebral Palsy is not the sole factor shaping the person I am today. The diagnosis itself is not what shapes a person, but rather the experiences they have and how those experiences imprint on them.

One interesting fact that many don't realize about having a primary disability is that they are often accompanied by the "gift" of one or multiple secondary conditions, which are directly related to the primary disabling condition. CP gifted me a severe gastrointestinal motility disorder that affects my entire digestive system, all the way from my esophagus to my rectum. This makes eating a blessing and a curse that often feels like a loathed chore. Food feels like my worst enemy most days. I eat and drink because I have to, because my body needs it, to function and survive.

Imagine sitting in bumper-to-bumper traffic not for minutes or hours, but for days or weeks; this is my digestive system. Heartburn, vomiting, and a bloated stomach that makes me look pregnant are just a few of the regular symptoms my body experiences.

I began experiencing symptoms at age 14 and was not accurately diagnosed until age 21. This led to me hearing over and over again, "It's in your head, and if you'd just learn to relax, you would be able to eat and go to the bathroom, like everyone else."

Ironically, when I received my correct diagnosis of Chronic Intestinal Pseudoobstruction (CIP), the doctor confirmed it WAS in my HEAD, but not the way others believed. My CP caused it, making my muscles and nerves in my digestive system unable to communicate, in the same way it affects other muscle groups and nerves in my body.

The difficulties with my digestive system are *real* and require my respect and attention to how, what, when, and the frequency of my eating to be comfortable and function productively.

In addition, I have something called Chronic Venous Insufficiency. The valves in my legs, responsible for helping push the blood up to my heart, do not work as they are meant to, causing the blood to pool in my legs and feet. Imagine a human being with feet the size of elephant's feet, making shoes that once fit comfortably, feel like a vice grip. Visualize trying to move your legs, which already seem to have a mind of their own, but cannot move an inch because your legs and feet feel like they have been cemented to the ground.

I know what you are thinking! My goodness, how many diagnoses does this woman have? That's the thing...

Here's what I've discovered. Every new symptom, brought on by a diagnois, led to another diagnosis. I was grateful to know what I was dealing with, don't get me wrong, but it seems that these diagnoses keep multiplying. Perhaps this is a fun place to add, I've actually not mentioned them all.

Everytime this happens, I'm expected to keep pushing-through. Those that say they support me, don't see that I now have added challenges, just that I better not "accept" these new limitations. I wish they would understand that my "accepting" does not mean I give in, it means I acknowledge this is what it is, so I can figure out how to keep thriving. If they would just **SEE ME**!

I AM: a daughter, a sibling, a niece, a cousin, an aunt, a friend, a dog lover, and a music lover.

My favorite genre is country music. However, I have an eclectic ear and palate for music, as I listen to most music genres. The criteria I use most of the time to decide whether I like a song are the melody of the music, and my ability to understand the lyrics/words being sung, because that is how I can connect, and be moved by the song.

I am a high school graduate, a college graduate, and a master's degree graduate. I have been an employee and an entrepreneur for the last 11 years. I am a Certified Personal Trainer and a Certified Life Coach.
I love nature, although it can be challenging to be in it as a full-time wheelchair user. However, I bring nature into my life by enjoying my backyard. I love to sit outside and feel the sun on my skin and face. I love to hear and feel a light breeze.

I have always thirsted for knowledge; I am a lifelong learner. Human nature and behavior have always fascinated me. From the time I was about 10 years old, my favorite genres of books were psychology, sociology, and self-help books. These books aimed to help me develop into the best version of myself that I could be, books that would help me understand myself, others, and how they behave, enhancing my ability to interact effectively with those around me.

The role I am most proud of is being a mom, and although it didn't start that way, I have been a single mom since my son was very young.

I am a fierce advocate for not only people with disabilities, but also all marginalized populations, aka underdogs. I fight for a world of full inclusion for all, where everyone can access every opportunity they wish to experience, without being prevented by physical and/or attitudinal barriers. The only thing that should stop anyone from experiencing something is that they decided it was not an experience they wanted to have a chance at.

I have hopes and dreams, have been defeated, and am victorious.
These are some of the ways I have been more than my diagnoses. I have turned lemons into sweet lemonade by turning "deficits" into missions and purpose. I learned to see what others call deficits as tremendous assets—assets meant to accomplish good in the world.

I am a deep thinker, problem-solver, analytical overthinker, and "recovering perfectionist." For years, I ended almost every spoken sentence with "I am sorry," as if I had to apologize for my thoughts and feelings, as a way to apologize for my very existence. Never again, I continue to show up as me, unapologetically, and I encourage and teach others how to do the same.

Have you ever felt like you got struck in the head by a lightning bolt? That's exactly how I felt when I realized that if I wanted others to see me the way I live, which is to be more than my diagnoses, I would have to be like a snake. I would have to shed my skin that has been hurt and damaged by the scars left by others. My new skin allows my true self to shine through. Whether or not my new skin is seen, is of no consequence to me. By keeping my focus on how I see myself, as more, helps others shift their gaze.

I laugh, I cry, I hurt, I dream, I bleed red. I am more like you than I am different.

Eleven years ago, when I started my life coaching business, I decided on the name Possibilities R Infinite. I recognized that there are an infinite number of possibilities for us all to experience and that we are not meant to experience them all. One can have infinite possibilities and experiences, and it is up to each person to choose which experiences they want.

However, to have a choice, they must have access to the experience so they can have the opportunity to experience it; without access, there is no experience.

Over a year ago, my personal and professional evolution led me to rebrand my business with Riseability™. Making this part of my vision, mission, and purpose seemed natural. RiseAbility is who I am every day, and it is part of the legacy I hope to leave in this world, upon my death.

To those reading this who live with a diagnosis—or who are simply navigating the hard days—I want you to know: you are more. You are allowed to be tired and brave, grieving and growing, hurting and hopeful.

You are not what others label you. You are not your lowest moment.

You are your resilience. You are your story. You are your strength.
So please, for the love of your own soul— Look past the frame... and
see you.

And when you look at me, don't just see the chair. Look past the frame
and see the person, the purpose, the fire, the possibility.

SEE ME.
"I ain't the less that some folks see, I'm a whole damn storm of ability.
So if you're lookin'—look deep and free; Look past the frame ... and
see me."

©Sharon Birn 4-19-25

BIO:

Sharon Birn is a certified personal trainer, certified coach, and a passionate disability advocate. As a multi-number-one international best-selling co-author and founder of Possibilities R Infinite and RiseAbility Fitness, Sharon aims to flip the label script and redefine how we see ability, strength, and potential.

Born with Cerebral Palsy and a full-time wheelchair user, Sharon has always been more than her diagnosis. Her Personal and professional experience has fueled a lifelong commitment to helping others rise—body, mind, and soul. Through her work with individuals with varying disabilities, physical limitations, seniors, and those recovering from injury, she proves that fitness and well-being are for everybody and EVERY BODY.

Sharon's philosophy centers on honoring the whole person and focusing on strengths rather than perceived deficits. Her RiseAbility approach energizes the body, elevates the mindset, and enhances independence. She believes that when we focus on what people can do, we ignite confidence, reduce self-doubt, and unlock true potential.

Sharon speaks, writes, and coaches to inspire a cultural shift that sees the woman sitting in the wheelchair before the chair itself. Her mission is clear: to spark a movement of inclusion, empowerment, and possibility where people of all abilities are seen, heard, and celebrated for the skills and gifts they bring.

www.linkedin.com/in/sharon-birn

www.possibilitiesrinfinite.com/home

DYING TO LIVE

by Nicole (Nic) Angai-Galindo

The ambiance while sitting here in my living room, about to write my chapter, is perfect. Fitting for the story to follow. In another hour or so, the moon will be up. The blinds are drawn now, earlier than usual. The shadows, being cast in the room from the one inch slits of light, coming through the vertical gaps in the blinds, loom behind me. I feel their eyes staring holes into the back of my neck. They are troubled by what I am about to share, for when I bring them into the light, they no longer exist.

I had to find a way to survive this again or lose everyone I loved, and all the ground I had covered, since the last time I fell to my knees. If I didn't, I feared that all the other times that I'd been here, one step closer to my death, would now be one time too many. Death was what awaited me, if I didn't find a way.

The soreness in the fleshy part of my palms lingered days after the incident, even though the redness had since disappeared. Staring at the ceiling fan whirling slowly above me, that horrific morning drive to work a week ago, played through slowly in my mind even slower than the sluggish movement of the ceiling fan.

A red light and the screeching of tires beside me shook me out of my daze. It did so thankfully, so that I could slam my foot on the brake. I wondered, as I glanced to my left, was the woman at the wheel in the car beside me watching her life crumble before her eyes as well? Did she feel it? Feel it coming? What was she going to do about it? I shivered. Was she really there or was the little voice being sucked down into the quicksand that was my logic, throwing out these questions to me?

When the light turned green, I pulled hurriedly over into the next street on my right. I stopped just shy of the edge of the driveway belonging to the last house on the cul de sac. Suddenly, my arms flew up into the air, grazing the cool vinyl ceiling of my truck. Just as suddenly, my arms crashed down. My palms hit the steering wheel so hard that I could feel the vibration up to my elbows. In a rhythmic movement, I kept repeating the rise and fall of my arms. Each time that my open palms hit the steering wheel I screamed, "Why me? Why Now? I can't do this again!"

I made it to work that day, ten minutes late, and with a third berating taken to my desk. I set it beside my other lateness souvenirs…

Dragging myself into a sitting position, I gingerly turned left and dropped my feet off the side of the bed. I needed to go to the bathroom. I needed to put the ceiling fan on a higher speed because I could feel the droplets of sweat running down the side of my left temple. I was making my way unsteadily to the corridor that led to the bathroom when I started retching. The disgusting tasting bile filled my mouth. Not wanting to spit it out and make another mess for my husband to clean up when he returned from work, I found the strength to dash to the bathroom.

Back to bed a few minutes later and again the floodgates flew open. This was my third mini-breakdown today. "Could a person really have multiple breakdowns in the span of just one day?" I thought to myself. The first one happened at 6:15AM as my husband was leaving for work. I didn't want him to go because I did not want to be alone. Yet, whenever he was at home, he was sitting perched on the edge of the bed at my side, simply holding my hands in his warm ones, staring intently at me while I said nothing.

My tummy was growling. I couldn't remember when was the last time that I ate something.

I could smell the spiciness of the roasting jalapenos in the air, my eyes slightly burning. I loved working in my in-laws Mexican restaurant with my husband. We were in the throes of COVID and I knew so many people were trapped in their homes. I felt lucky to be able to have somewhere to go every day. We served takeout, over a table set up at the front door.

How funny that I was working in a Spanish restaurant. Me, a Trinidadian-born woman, trying to recall the five years of this foreign language that I'd mastered enough to get an outstanding grade upon high school graduation.

Months later, when I did return to my full-time office job, I would still work at the restaurant part-time. Well, it was full-time hours around a part-time schedule. Between the two jobs I was putting in four sixteen hour days a week and two twelve hour days on the weekend. I was happily exhausted until that exhaustion caught up to me, forcing me on a downward spiral.

It was a slow spiral that began with me trying to hold on, digging my fingernails into the surface of reality.

I lost the battle.

On my way down, I caught glimpses of the empty antidepressant bottles rolling around at the back of the top drawer in the bathroom vanity. I heard the clinking of the empty beer bottles stuffed into doubled thirteen gallon drawstring plastic bags, as I snuck out the front door to take them to the garbage cans at the side of the house.

Friday's five and Saturday's six plus the doubles on a weeknight after reaching home at 11PM. I had been drinking about a case of beer plus, a week.

Legs swung off the side of the bed for the second time today, I dragged my feet going into the kitchen. I opened the refrigerator. Of course there was no beer in it. When I crashed, my husband popped the cap off of each bottle of beer that was left in the refrigerator and poured the bitter, golden liquid down the drain.

To this day I still crave that first icy sip from the salt rimmed bottle on a scorching Summer day.

It is Summer now and I know that one of these upcoming weekends, I will have to fight back the urge. Yet after the second sip, I'm so turned off.

I reached into the refrigerator and removed a vanilla flavored yogurt. It seemed that I could only get down non-solids these days. Smoothies, jello, and soup made up my diet for the last three weeks. "Tomorrow is

Saturday." I thought "Or is it?" I'd lost track of which day of the week it was. If so, then our telehealth call was at 9AM. 'Our' telehealth call because my husband participated in these each week, wanting to hear what my psychiatrist had to say about the progress he reported.

I certainly didn't feel as if any progress were being made. Have you ever felt that no matter how hard you are trying, you aren't getting anywhere? I felt as if I were swimming with all my upper body strength, against the strongest current which was only keeping me in the same spot.

That evening, after my husband returned from work, he got me out of my robe and into a tee and jogging pants. He had to double knot the drawstring after cinching in the waistband because the pants were sliding off my skinny hips. He half dragged, half carried me, to the back porch and gently eased me into our rocking chair. The one that he had in the bedroom of his apartment when we were dating. The one I would rock back and forth in while imitating rowing a boat and singing row, row, row your boat. Then we would look at each other and both burst out laughing.

Where had that woman gone? It seemed that every now and then over the last forty four years of my life I would lose her.

As the third week rolled into the forth, I slowly started gaining my strength back. The combination of medication that I had been prescribed was working its way back into my system. Two antidepressants, Celexa and Wellbutrin, plus a mood stabilizer, Lamotragine. My appetite slowly started returning and I could keep down some solids. Every day my sister would call on her lunch break to see how I was doing. We would chat for ten or fifteen minutes and then I would go back and lay down.

An hour or so later, I would get back up and sit on the couch which faced the sliding doors that opened onto the back porch. Just a week ago, I would not draw the blinds. Now I did. I sat at a folding dinner table, building a puzzle from the dollar store. This became my weekday routine. By the time my two month short-term disability came to an end, I had pieced together three five-hundred piece puzzles and completed a fifteen hundred piece one, that I had started a month before I fell apart. It seemed that building puzzles was the only thing that distracted me from the emptiness in my brain, the numbness in my heart. Even so, a turmoil of emotions crawled along the surface of my skin incessantly.

One morning, a few weeks later I gathered up our dirty laundry into the three plastic color coordinated baskets, loaded them into our pickup, and sent my husband a text message that I was going to the laundromat. He immediately dialed back and when I answered, I knew he knew that I was going to be ok.

Those were the longest two months of our lives. I had lived the nightmare before, with others, who would not be able to withstand the bipolar blow that I was dealt, every time I misstepped or for whatever reason, the universe seemed bored and needed to get a hoot out of messing with my head.

Do you know what it feels like to go from feeling so afraid and helpless that you would not take a shower unless your husband were sitting on the closed toilet seat waiting for you, to get back behind the wheel after two months of not driving? You may never have lived this exact scenario but I bet that every single one of you have felt both powerless at times and then empowered again.

The sad truth is that I had seen it coming. It was not my first ferris wheel ride. I knew that with the controls unmanned every top of ride would not result in a seamless 180 to the bottom of ride. I knew that unmanned it would feel like the most twisted, fearsome, heart-plunging roller coaster ever built... and I hated rides. Knowing that never stopped me from jumping on the damn ride before, but this time was the worst. A few days on the ride was one thing. Eight weeks, a whole other story.

Two months before I went out on STD, my husband had lost his job due to COVID. He started a new job two weeks after I had to run away from mine. We cleaned out our modest savings, and the disability check, a whopping $171 a week, just about covered the psychiatrist's fee without medical benefits. The $50 left over each week went toward my medication.

A combination of working myself almost to death, self medicating with alcohol, and being irresponsible about managing my bipolar medicine, almost cost me my life. Again. Though drinking had not been a part of the mix before, overworking myself was nothing new to me.

Strangely, I haven't completed a puzzle since. I have saved them all however. My husband carefully taped them all at the back and one of them sits on my desk at work now. The big one. The fifteen hundred piece one. A reminder yes, of a period in my life where ill-made and oftentimes ill-fitting puzzle pieces, purchased for a buck for 500 saved my life. They kept my hands moving, and my mind thinking, while the medication my brain needed did its thing.

"Life is like a box of chocolates." - Forrest Gump.

Or, is it like a puzzle?

"Life is like a puzzle." - Nic, the Gifted Bipolar Writer

Each piece is not meant to be placed until it's time. You will spot the pieces and it may convey something to you, though you don't know what just yet. Perhaps it's a bit of color that will catch your eye, the curve of an outline, the shadow on a piece of white but until that piece is meant to be placed, it will not fit. The picture will not become clear until all of the pieces are placed. I held onto building those puzzles during that time. I know now it was as a way to maintain control; control over something when everything else around me, or rather, within me, was spinning out of control.

Once I took back control of my life (with the help of medication and talk-therapy), the universe knew better than to mess with me.

That last fall, the one I had to forgive myself for so that I could heal, was in 2020. On July 1st of 2021 we purchased our first home. A year later, my husband, who was brought to the USA by his parents when he was five years old, and who had lived here his whole life trying to attain legal status, got his green card. Today, he is a naturalized American citizen.

The job that I returned to after my two month absence, the one where on the first day of my return I was sat down in the conference room and told by the vice president, to never discuss what happened with any of my co-workers, is now history. I'd been to hell and back and I'd be damned if the person that signed my paycheck felt that he owned my life enough, that he could tell me what I could and could not share with others.

I've spent the last few years living a life of gratitude. Finding joy in the simple things, like savoring a good cup of coffee while sitting on the back stoop, looking onto our beautiful backyard. It's surrounded by trees on the perimeter but flat for the two hundred feet it extends to the wooded area at the back, where the deer like to wander in from and nibble at whatever it is they seem to feast on.

The day after this book launch, July 5th, will be the second year anniversary with my company. I walked into this one wearing my bipolarness on my sleeve. Like my boss says, "Nicole is a storm system, you have to see what's coming before it hits." They know who I am, where my heart is; they give me the space and the grace I need when I need it. As a result, my focus and my work are one hundred times what it's ever been.

I will never again hide who I am from anyone. I will never again ignore the whispered voice that I know belongs to me and the almost imperceptible message it carries. Imperceptible because of all the noise of the world around me drowning it out.

You must stay in tune to the pitch of that whisper. You must trust it to guide you and stop and heed what it's telling you. Your very life depends on it. Mine did and because I didn't heed it, I almost lost it.

We all have the survival instinct within us but that does not guarantee that we will all survive. In fact, some will never again step into the light because they have lived in the dark for too long. Sharing my story has helped many people to understand that we must first embrace that which we think is so wrong with us, as the very thing that can be so right about us. It is the thing that pushes us to take the broken pieces and make ourselves whole again.

And, once you are whole again, you will want nothing more than to help others bring their shadows into the light, so they no longer exist.

Are you ready to step into the light?

This chapter, with minor alterations, was written by me in 2024, and was published with another publisher July 4th, 2024. Almost a year to the date that this book: WE CHOOSE TO BE MORE THAN OUR DIAGNOSES, my vision, and now as a publisher myself, is published on July 1st, 2025.

My hope is that after reading my chapter you see the passing of time, and how living in faith and not fear, can change what appears to be one's fate.

BIO:

Nicole Angai-Galindo, aka Nic, is on a mission to show the world that having a mental illness does not determine the level of happiness and success that one can achieve in life. She is known to many on her social media platform of choice, LinkedIn, as The Gifted Bipolar Writer. She has co-authored eleven Best-Selling Anthologies, starting in 2023. Five of these were published by her. In February of 2025, Nic left her full-time job and established Guiding Briliant Writers Publishing, LLC. Born in Trinidad & Tobago, in the Caribbean, she migrated to the U.S. at 19 years old with $100 in her pocket and a suitcase full of clothes. She often jokes that she is made in the U.S. with Trini parts. She's a devoted wife and proud mom who now lives in New York.

www.linkedin.com/in/nicthegbw
www.amazon.com/Note-My-Family-Your-Legacy

Photo Description:

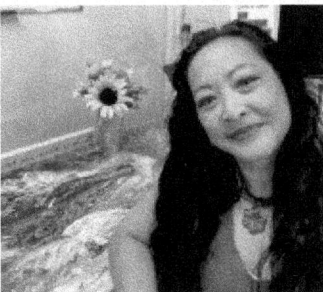

Nic at her desk in work with the 1500 piece puzzle she talks about in her story. The ornamental plaque on her desk behind the puzzle, is a souvenir she picked up a year after her short-term disability, during a trip to Canada to visit her sister.

It reads, "She believed she could, so she did."

www.ingramcontent.com/pod-product-compliance
Lightning Source LLC
Chambersburg PA
CBHW051825090426
42736CB00011B/1659